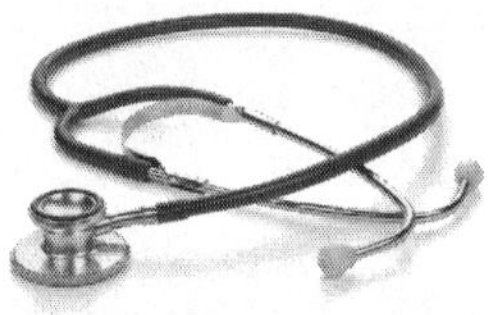

PRAISE FOR WAYNE LIEBHARD'S OTHER BOOKS

THE VORTEX EFFECT

The Vortex Effect is intelligent, compelling, and fun. Laced with the keen observations of a first-rate physician, the irreverence of a life-long musician, and the musings of a serious wonk, Vortex takes aim at almost all of contemporary America's sacred cows, with humor, passion and suspense.

– Elinor Burkett—Oscar winner and New York Times best-selling author

Dr. Wayne Liebhard has seen the best and the worst of American medicine, music and politics. And he'd like to see a few things changed! Thank goodness he's created Derek Mann to share his ideas with us. Equal parts drama, social commentary, and metaphysical exploration, Mann's story, at heart, is every person's search for happiness and meaning in a society that wants to paint us all the same shade of gray. This book is bound to stimulate conversations long after readers have put it down. Bravo!

–Dr. Ann Korbel—Editor

The Vortex Effect is a riveting adventure. It grabs your attention and sucks you into a remarkable twisting, turning suspense tale, while simultaneously forcing you to question the boundaries of your own existence. Wayne Liebhard's protagonist, Dr. Derek Mann, is the perfect conduit for the trip, and this ride will leave you permanently changed. I especially enjoyed the music theme that runs through the book. One gets the feeling that Dr. Mann would rather be on stage playing his guitar than in the ER.

– Jim Donna of The Castaways—
Co-author of Liar, Liar. Member Minnesota
Rock & Country Hall of Fame

If you find it hard to believe the doctor you've come to enjoy, and think you know, is much more than a white coat learning digital record keeping, then you must read *The Vortex Effect*. If you've worked every day with a doctor who has an extraordinary affection for his undergrad alma mater, and will do great rock 'n' roll after just two beers, then get ready for a real ER doc having a mind-altering experience in Wayne Liebhard's *The Vortex Effect*.

– Dave Durenberger U.S. Senator (R-MN)
1978-95 St. John's University '55

Dr. Wayne Liebhard's most recent novel, *The Vortex Effect*, is a fascinating combination of a strange internal experience combined with a unique mystery. Dr. Liebhard is a respected physician who shows great perception about what ails health care in 2015. This is a well written novel that rivets one's attention and is very hard to put down.

– Thomas A. Stolee, M.D.—past president,
Minnesota Medical Association

ELEPHANTS IN THE EXAM ROOM

Elephants in The Exam Room is a powerful book. The author, Dr. Wayne Liebhard, picks apart the American health care system and shows why we are in a health care crisis and what needs to be done about it. What I found extraordinary about this book is that Liebhard not only candidly exposes the problems within America's health care system, but he also offers realistic and practical solutions. I hope every American reads this book and voices their concern, even outrage, at what's going on.

– Karen Coiffi-Ventrice of BookPleasures.com

Health care is a very touchy and complicated subject, so let me refer you to what I think is the best treatise I have ever read on this subject: *Elephants in the Exam Room* by Dr. Wayne Liebhard.

– Minnesota State Representative Michael Beard

While I was in the U.S. Senate trying to change the practice of medicine by changing the way Medicare finances patient care, Wayne and doctors like him were growing frustrated. First in their efforts to meet patient needs and demands, and then by the changes in the system, in the life styles of practitioners, and the growing emphasis by folks like me in changing practice behavior from the outside in. For those of us who believe that community and family health professionals, not bionic medicine men, are the key to improved access, quality, and cost, this nicely-written plea by a Minnesota doc and friend is a good read.

– Former U.S. Senator Dave Durenberger,
Director, National Institute of Health Policy

Elephants in The Exam Room is a warning to patients and a wake-up call to physicians. With a blunt tongue and a few pointed fingers, Dr. Liebhard debunks health care myths and demystifies the dangerous doublespeak of today's health care debate. Every reader should heed Dr. Liebhard's warning before there are only elephants left in the room, and no doctors to be found.

– Twila Brase, RN, PHN,
President, Citizen's Council on Health Care

This book is a "must-read" for anyone interested in returning control of their health care decisions to consumers and their physicians, and away from government regulators and HMO executives.

–Thomas A. Stolee, M.D., Past President,
Minnesota Medical Association

These books are available at wayneliebhard.com.

WORKS BY WAYNE LIEBHARD

Fiction

The Vortex Effect

Nonfiction

Elephants in The Exam Room (The Big Picture Solution To Today's Health Care "Crisis") 2009

Elephants in The Exam Room (The Seven Things You Need To Know About Today's Health Care "Crisis") 2007

Walking The Tightrope —Trusting Your Life To Telemedicine

Music (Available through all major streaming sites)

Here—In Flyover Country (Original Album)

I like Livin' Here (Original Album)

No Rules (Original Album)

Reflections (Original Album)

Music Videos

For The Solid Gold Band

WALKING THE TIGHTROPE–TRUSTING YOUR LIFE TO TELEMEDICINE

LESSONS FROM EARLY IN THE COVID-19 PANDEMIC

Wayne D. Liebhard, M.D.

Alethos Press - Woodbury MN

Alethos Press, Woodbury MN – https://alethospress.com

Walking the Tightrope–Trusting Your Life to Telemedicine

ISBN:

Print: 978-0-9863773-9-6
Digital: 979-8-9863314-0-9

Printed in the U.S. by Bethany Press International

Cover Design by Sammi Griffin Art

Graphic and Layout Services by Dave Racer, MLitt

https://wayneliebhard.com/

First Printing

PRAISE FOR *WALKING THE TIGHTROPE*

We are living in a world where, for many, convenience seems to trump reasoning when it comes to choosing medical care. Patients demand it, and corporate medical America is happy to supply it – hastened by the government-sponsored expansion of telemedicine.

Dr. Wayne Liebhard's new book *Walking The Tightrope – Trusting Your Life To Telemedicine* is a stark wake-up call to those who believe that their doctors may still be in a position to regulate the safety of telemedicine for acute care.

This book is a must-read for all consumers of medical care, as the inside information it provides on how we got here – and how we can use that information to forge a safer future – is invaluable.

– David Durenberger,
Former United States Senator and
Director of National Institute of Health Policy

Walking The Tightrope carefully examines the pressures that doctors face as they strive to provide safe and appropriate health care. It also examines how the practice of medicine arrived at this place where third parties decide what is best for a patient instead of the physician and patient working together. Dr. Liebhard offers a way to use this knowledge to chart a safe path forward.

We live in a time when many Americans tend to believe that any good or service they choose to consume has been rigorously tested for safety. Patients also believe their physicians are free to make independent decisions about the best and most appropriate medical care in each instance. Are either of these assumptions true?

– Dave Racer, MLitt
Publisher, writer and author of
21 books about health care

During the Covid-19 pandemic, physicians and patients switched to doing virtual telemedicine visits rather than in-person clinical appointments. Telemedicine can be a good thing for improving patient access to medical professionals. But there are important caveats, as Dr. Liebhard explains.

In today's corporate medical culture, physicians are directed by their employers as a business decision to provide virtual visits. But virtual visits are clearly not the same as in-person medical consultations. Liebhard gets to the point: "Who wouldn't trust a large medical conglomerate that owns hospitals and all sorts of shiny new multiple story buildings when they advertise their telemedicine services with the following: 'get the same great care as with an office visit?'"

This question leads to Dr. Liebhard's *tour de force* argument for earning and maintaining trusted and trusting doctor-patient relationships. Today the doctor is usually employed by a mega hospital-clinic organization. But Liebhard says: “A physician should never allow herself or himself to work *for the corporation*. Physicians should always work *for their patients*.”

The good news: Patients can actively query their doctors about who they are working for. After all, they are trained to serve patients and do no harm, and that's why they became physicians. The book includes an illuminating interview with internist Dr. Donald Gehrig who describes a successful and fulfilling direct pay primary care practice, and a history of how corporate medicine was spawned in Minnesota.

I highly recommend this book.

-- Lee Beecher, M.D. (Em).
Dr. Beecher is the co-author of *Passion for Patients*, (2021) Alethos Press.

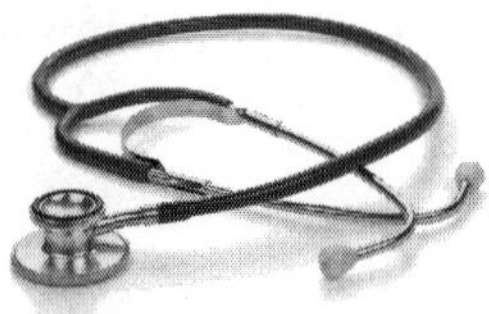

TABLE OF CONTENTS

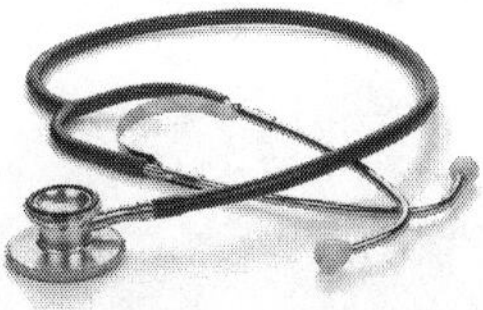

Dedication

To all my patients–past, present, and future.

ACKNOWLEDGMENTS

The mechanics of writing a book may boil down to the individual efforts of an author, but the substance of the result is composed of many diverse ingredients, including some borrowed from the experiences and insights of others.

I am blessed to be able to tap into an incredible network of individuals who remain uninhibited in expressing their insights on the world, and who remain equally open to subjecting those results to critique. To them, I offer deep gratitude.

My deepest gratitude is reserved for my wife Joy, who most closely interacted with me during the process of simultaneously practicing medicine and writing another book. I cannot find a way to better describe her profound influence than to co-opt the words of Jerome Groopman, fellow physician and author of *How Doctors Think*. As Dr. Groopman notes, "It is a gift to live your life with a person you love who is wiser than you." While I often give myself credit for the ability to see the "big picture," Joy reminds me again and again how to move the chaff out of the way to get there.

Special thanks to my agent, Liz Trupin-Pulli, whose developmental editing skills were essential in refining the message this book was intended to convey. Thanks also to those who offered their personal experiences and insight, especially best-selling author Elinor Burkett, Dr. Donald Gehrig, MD, Senator Dave Durenberger, and legendary musician Jim Donna. Also, to my patients, thanks for the many years of being allowed to assist in preserving healthy lives, and for being an impetus to fight for the sanctity of the doctor-patient relationship.

Alethos Press and it's CEO Dave Racer have also been a special blessing in their ability to value the uncloaking of issues that, to some, may appear controversial. Many thanks!

If indeed the truth will set us free, then let us strive to proclaim it.

FOREWORD

By Dave Racer, MLitt

When today's physicians still practicing medicine started their careers in the 1980s, the world (and the practice of medicine) was vastly different. Many physicians admit to feeling betrayed in that the current practice of medicine is "not what I signed up for." Are they right? And if so, doesn't everything change? Or is this a matter of whether every change is good for patients—and physicians?

Doctors knew that they weren't signing up for short hours, mega salaries, or easy work. They signed up to be trained to use their skills to make decisions to reduce their patients' pain and suffering and extend the patient's life when possible. As a doctor, they hoped to offer patients a better life. Some physicians knew that they weren't well-suited for the ladder-climbing milieu of the business world. Indeed, the idea of working independently motivated them.

Working independently with a patient, physicians knew, would be welded to taking a serious responsibility for the patient's welfare. Physicians believe that clinical safety and appropriateness are ensured when decisions affecting patients, especially those resulting in life or death, are made through a doctor-patient alliance, without undue outside influence. Doctors accepted this responsibility for patient outcomes contingent on their ability to "practice without their hands being tied."

Practicing independently in each patient's best interest is precisely what physicians "signed up for" and what today, many lament. Corporate and government intrusion into their independent practice of medicine over the last five decades has left physicians saddled with an impossible task of trying to maintain their oath and their responsibility to patients while simultaneously being stripped of their ability to do so.

Since the early 1990s, Dr. Wayne Liebhard has written and lectured about the dangers of third-party interference with the physician's practice of medicine. He is deeply alarmed about the newest promise to "revolutionize" medicine—over-reliance on telemedicine as a panacea to improve medical care.

Dr. Liebhard, as a practicing physician, knows that some forms of medical care are appropriate for some patients, while a different approach works for others. He practices the "art" of medicine. The idea of over-relying on telemedicine highly concerns him. There is a time and place for it, but only when appropriate.

Hence, *Walking The Tightrope – Trusting Your Life To Telemedicine* is not a blanket condemnation of the use of telemedicine. Telemedicine – when used properly – can be a useful arrow in the quiver of diagnostic options open to physicians. Physicians, however, need to decide – along with their patients – when telemedicine is safe and appropriate.

Government-sponsored expansion of the use of telemedicine services during the early Covid-19 pandemic, unfortunately, has led to the promotion of its use to attempt to treat almost any condition imaginable – sometimes with tragic results.

What if telemedicine is not safe, or appropriate, to evaluate a patient's abdominal pain, elevated temperature, or seriousness of what otherwise seems a minor or benign issue? Does a patient know – in today's world of corporate and government dominated health care – whether the doctor is recommending or even requiring a telemedicine visit because he or she believes it is safe and appropriate, or because the corporation he or she works for requires it?

Walking The Tightrope carefully examines the pressures that doctors face as they strive to provide safe and appropriate health care. It also examines how the practice of medicine arrived at this place where third parties decide what is best for a patient instead of the physician and patient working together. Dr. Liebhard offers a way to use this knowledge to chart a safe path forward.

We live in a time when many Americans tend to believe that any good or service they choose to consume has been rigorously tested for safety. Patients also believe their physicians are free to make independent decisions about the best and most appropriate medical care in each instance. Are either of these assumptions true?

Don't bet on it.

-- Dave Racer, MLitt, is a publisher, editor, and author with more than 20 books about medical care and health care finance to his credit. Learn more about Mr. Racer at https://daveracer.com

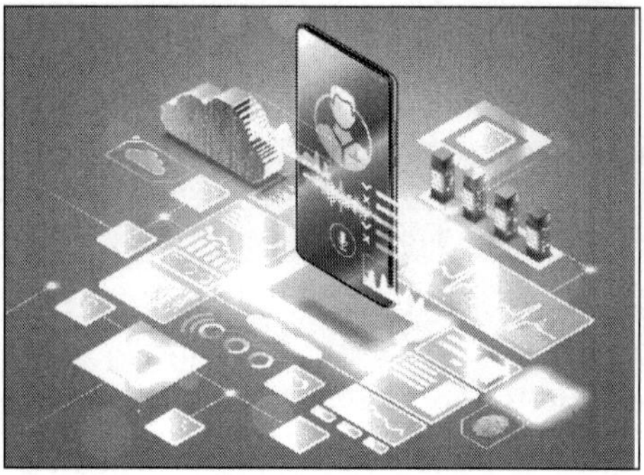

"As desires drive a society's changes, they don't necessarily drive it's best interests..."

– Wayne Liebhard, M.D.

"If you find a path with no obstacles, it probably doesn't lead anywhere."

– Frank A. Clark

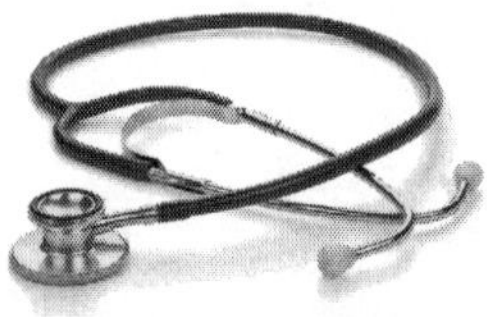

Introduction

Imagine this scenario: An elderly gentleman is undergoing a video visit with a physician. He is somewhat confused, and the history of his concern comes from his wife and from him. He says the symptoms of his buttocks and rectal pain have been present for one day. She says three days, but they both say the pain is severe and has worsened. The pain is the worst when he moves. He describes fevers, but this being a video visit, no vital signs were taken.

He is observed to be lying comfortably in bed – which is the extent of the "physical exam." He is prescribed a muscle relaxant for likely muscle spasm, and counseled about the medication. No other specific warnings or follow-up information is given.

The next day the patient presents to the clinic because he is unable to urinate. He is found to have an extremely low blood pressure and is immediately hospitalized and found to have necrotizing fasciitis – flesh eating bacteria – forcing him to undergo multiple surgical procedures to remove decayed and infected tissues in an attempt to save his life, unsuccessfully.

The early days of the Covid-19 pandemic knocked the practice of American medicine off its feet. The ensuing government promotion of expanded telemedicine services helped alleviate access issues created by the pandemic. It also opened the door for the astonishing use of telemedicine for just about any medical condition imaginable – which should scare the hell out of anyone who is interested in continuing to receive consistently high-quality medical care for acute conditions. Presented here is an analysis of those days, how we got there, and what they taught us about forging a safe path forward – for everyone.

Welcome to the new age of telemedicine – the next great promise in the delivery of medical care. Yet another revolution that will undoubtedly "save" health care in the United States. Indeed, Doctors Ezekiel Emanuel and Amal Navathe of the Healthcare Transformation Institute at the University of Pennsylvania list it as one of the "three major changes that have been the anticipated silver lining of Covid – 19." In their April 14, 2020 article in the New York Times, "Will 2020 Be the Year That Medicine Was Saved?," they note that "telemedicine is cost-effective for matters that do not need physical contact and easier to work into patients' daily life, and it frees up office visits for patients with complex conditions."

In principle, it is hard to disagree with the last statement as it relates to some conditions and to some specialty care – those for which telemedicine may be appropriate. In clinical reality, recall the patient we just mentioned (we'll call him "George") – someone you might encounter when taking a trip from the ivory tower to the trenches. Should George have had physical contact at his initial visit – or at least have been immediately referred for it? Given that he died, and that more rapid proper diagnosis and treatment may have saved his life, the answer is obvious. Should George's complaint have been "seen" at all through a video visit? That answer is also obvious.

George's doctor worked for a corporation – a corporation that decided how its doctors would employ a telemedicine platform to treat its patients. In itself, does this imply that medical corporations are inherently malicious? No, it does not, but it does imply that corporations are interested in the treatment of populations. Conversely, doctors are trained primarily to think about, and to treat, individuals. The intersection of these inclinations is where the rubber meets the road, and where it may be determined if you as a patient get safely to your destination, or if you get run over. As for the ivory tower – by all means, let them weigh in on the issue, as long as they remember the answer to the age-old question: "What's the difference between God and a doctor?" Answer: "God doesn't think he's a doctor."

Is telemedicine the next "fix" in line, or the next debacle? While medical ethicists need to continue to examine the big picture, trench dwellers such as myself need to sound the early alarms. Without these alarms, we remain subject to the risk that experimental trends can lead to entrenched, unintended-consequence realities. Without these alarms, and without the inside knowledge of why we sound them, patients like George may become lost to their families. Hence, this book. Oversight is an essential endeavor, especially in today's medical world. Here, I'll co-opt and slightly modify a phrase often attributed to Thomas Jefferson: "The price of medical freedom is eternal vigilance." That vigilance, however, is a two-way street. Patients who decide for themselves that the major determinant of good health care is an increasing level of convenience should not labor under the impression that the risks associated with their choices are somehow always being abated by their health care "providers."

Such is the case with telemedicine. Many of my colleagues and I are not concerned so much about using telemedicine in general (despite what the "doctors refuse to adapt" crowd spouts) as we are about the type of "care" we are often being coerced to provide in its use. Physicians have a moral and ethical duty to their patients to provide care that is safe and appropriate, despite outside pressures that may push them elsewhere. The goal of this book is to examine the current pressures and issues with telemedicine, along with the corporate and government influences behind those pressures – especially as they relate to a push toward an almost unbridled use of telemedicine to provide urgent/acute care medical services. As we progress, the massive reach of corporate and government control of the current practice of medicine will be obvious.

I dearly love the state of Minnesota, but as a practicing primary care physician in the Twin Cities area for over thirty-five years, I've endured more supposed "fixes" to medicine than anyone should be forced to suffer – most of which never really panned out and some of which led to painful unintended consequences. I've endured the fixes as a family physician doing hospital work including obstetrics, as a specialty occupational medicine practitioner, in working ERs and working as a hospitalist, and the last 18 years in an urgency room type setting. I'll ask you to pardon me from the onset if – after this many years of attempted fixes – I appear suspect as hell about yet another corporate and government attempt to "revolutionize" medicine.

What has formed my frame of reference is outlined in one of my earlier books, *Elephants in the Exam Room – The Big Picture Solution To Today's Health Care "Crisis."* "Minnesota is a place that healthcare executives like to refer to as the 'cradle of innovation' for healthcare, while many of my primary-care physician colleagues refer to it as the 'cesspool of practice.' My time here has given me a rather unique perspective that includes over three decades of weathering changes in the hotbed of managed-care experimentation, where most everything that comes your way in the rest of the United States seems to get its start." (See also: "The Minnesota Experience" and "Health Care Costs" in the appendix to this book.) While some of the concerns related to the expansion of telemedicine have Minnesota roots, telemedicine's almost unbridled expansion is most certainly a national issue, and we will be examining input on the issue from experts across the country.

What's my stake in this game? I can assure you that I personally am not anti-corporate, anti-management, or against any ethical means by which to deliver high-quality medical care at a reasonable cost. I'm not sitting on anyone's board, endorsing anyone's product, or running for office. Believe it or not, I'd just like to see all of us stay safe when we access medical care. Sad to say, in today's world, some areas of medical care have become a bit of a minefield, requiring pertinent background information for safe navigation. Sometimes that requires pointing out stark reality. Sometimes that requires calling out entities whose bottom line appears more important than their "covered lives." Sometimes that means calling out politicians who promote less than safe medical care practices because they appear to be a quick "fix" to cost and access issues, even when their "emergency" use ends. This book will not avoid those tasks, especially as we now see the statement: "I trust American medicine," get increasingly replaced by the question: "How do I trust American medicine?"

To get to what I define in Chapter One as "optimum care" it is necessary to understand the above influences and use that knowledge to chart our best course for medical care. Keeping that in mind, Chapter Two poses the central question: "Who Controls the Narrative and the Delivery of Care?" followed by a look at the role of technology on medicine in general (and on telemedicine in specific) in Chapter Three.

At some point in our lives, we are all patients, and now more than ever it is imperative that we understand the outside forces that influence decision-making in medical care. Once we understand who controls the narrative, we can understand who is really in charge of medical care decision- making. When we understand who is really in charge of that decision-making, we can then chart the best healthcare course for ourselves as individuals.

Patients today still largely believe that their primary care doctors are free to make the best unencumbered choices for their individual healthcare. While that may be the standard we desire, it is not a consistent reality. Corporate and government control over your physician is a concept that is not easy to accept. As we proceed I promise you to be blunt, to the point, and to protect no one when it comes to describing the landscape that consumers of medical care are driving into – or should I say, looking at on a screen. (There will also be no attempt to avoid humor as we do it.) We will be examining a number of different viewpoints from the literature – presented as information to consumers of health care (all of us) who may choose (or be pushed toward the use of) telemedicine (Chapter Four).

It's important to note that I'm not here to tell patients to second-guess their doctors. I am here to tell them to find a doctor who is willing to, when necessary, second-guess the system that he or she may work in. That, admittedly, is not always easy. In fact, it's never easy, especially if you work in a large healthcare system. Doctors have the reality of families to consider and bills to pay, just like everyone else. They nonetheless are obliged to adhere to their oath, which first and foremost demands that they do no harm. (Chapter 5 – What's Worse Than No Diagnosis?)

Regarding large healthcare systems, Doctors Emanuel and Navathe assert that one of the policies that government should adopt is that medical practices should be supported if they stay independent. Again, I can't disagree, in principle. However, that horse is already out of the barn here and by now has probably trotted somewhere into the southern hemisphere. As of 2018, less than one third of medical practices in the United States remained independent – a number that drops precipitously by the year. This unfortunately means that giving the finger to your health care system these days about care practices over which you disagree – as gallant as it sounds – may also mean that your other fingers have nowhere else to work. Our oath as physicians, however, demands that Doctor Nero does not sit idly by while Rome burns.

My personal recourse toward sanity as I continue to practice medicine has been to sound the alarm regarding the erosion of the doctor-patient relationship as loudly as I can (Chapter 6). Writing books, articles, and lecturing has indeed been cathartic for me, and perhaps has helped dent a relentless juggernaut seemingly intent on hijacking the practice of medicine.

Many long-term physicians know that the practice of medicine is being hijacked. As hijacking in general goes, if you're plane gets hijacked, you may end up landing in Miami instead of Dallas. You may also end up crash landing in the middle of a cornfield. We would – of course – never board a plane when we were convinced there was a high likelihood that its final stop would be a bed of cornstalks. Should we feel any differently about boarding the medical plane, or do we just hop on, convinced that we won't crash because our doctors are always following the principle of "do no harm?"

"Do no harm" implies that our clinicians are not intending to cause harm – but does it imply that they are fully attempting to avoid the potential for harm? The difference here may seem subtle, but it's not. For a Minnesota guy, it's kind of like driving your buddy over frozen ice during one of our winters to get to your fishing house. (Yeah, we're a bit crazy up here.) Obviously, no one is intending to have their vehicle break through the ice, but, for the sake of your buddy, have you attempted to avoid harm by actually checking the thickness of the ice yourself? (Chapter 7 – "Minimizing The Fallout" – is a guideline for the avoidance of harm.) Or, are you just relying on the fact that someone told you (or suggested) that the ice was safe?

It is the same with every piece of advice your doctor gives you and every action he or she takes. You are the passenger in the car your doctor is driving over the ice, and you've put your trust in the person behind the wheel. Why is it that you assume that the good doctor has indeed checked the thickness of the ice? The flashing letters "M. D." on the dashboard? The fact that the "car" is a brand-spanking-new five-story office building? The fact that your friend Stacey said she rode across the ice with him and all went well?

It could be any one, or all of the above, that convinced you to take that ride. Good news is, you will almost always arrive at your fishing spot safely. Bad news is, when you don't, the consequence is not a crappy plate of pasta because you chose the wrong restaurant. It's a watery grave. The specialized training that doctors and airline pilots and train conductors have isn't for 95% of the trips. It's for the 5% of the time or less when there is an unknown thin spot in the ice – where training, knowledge, and the wherewithal to handle the situation saves lives.

OK – all fine and good (and I'm running out of metaphors). So – where is the problem? You found a doctor you feel you can trust to do no harm and away you go across the ice.

Back up the train for a minute. (Sorry – not quite out of metaphors – and certainly not done mixing them.) Here's where the real questions start. Let's go back to our patient George. Was George's doctor intending to do any harm? Quite the contrary, actually. "Do no harm" implies not intending to do harm. But, how do you know if your doctor has gone further – and is attempting to avoid the potential for harm? As you make the trip across the ice, do you trust that your doctor has made certain the ice is safe?

Our patient George did. He and his wife deemed the ice of telemedicine to be safe. Why? Because they knew it was safe, or because they trusted it to be safe since their doctor was using it? Did they do their own research – i.e., did they drill their own holes in the ice to check its thickness? Do they own an ice auger – i.e., are they capable? Should they even have to own an ice auger – or should they reasonably expect that someone should have drilled holes for them?

Fact is, today's medical care-consuming public is overwhelmingly convinced that someone should drill the holes for them, and, indeed, that those holes are regularly being drilled.

Don't bet on it.

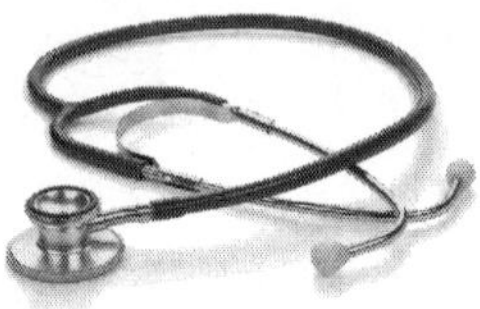

Chapter One

What Is Optimum Medical Care?

There is nothing quite like starting out with a question that is difficult, if not impossible, to adequately answer. Nonetheless, it is a question that needs to be posed, and an attempt needs to be made at an answer. Why? Because the entire endeavor of providing medical care – like so many other services – is geared toward providing not only what consumers desire, but also to provide what is best for them – the optimum. Perhaps nowhere today, other than in the delivery of medical care, is the definition of "optimum" more divergent than it is between the providers and consumers of that care.

While studies still seem to suggest that patients rank interpersonal interactions with their caregivers at the top of their list when it comes to medical care, the rest of that list has changed dramatically in recent years, most notably in relation to the notion of "convenience." Consumers of medical care, henceforth referred to as "patients," still desire competent, empathetic, affordable medical care. Just as importantly now, they also want the provision of that care to fit their lifestyles – in other words, they want it fast and easy, as well as being inexpensive. Like everything else in America, though, "fast and easy" is never supposed to imply "risky and unpredictable." Kind of like that hamburger from McDonald's. Why? Because there is always someone in America looking out for the welfare of the consumer of everything commercially branded, correct?

Anyone with half a functioning brain understands the potential risk in buying five pounds of shrimp on a 90-degree day from some guy selling it off the back of his rusty pickup truck. The sign for "Jim and Bob's Bungee Jumping/Go-Cart Track/Hog Roast" establishment should likewise get you to think critically about whether you should exit I-95 to check it out. For most anything else in America, we have a vast array of consumer protection agencies, oversight bureaus, and government commissions to ensure that anything we touch, consume, or breathe in should always be free from harm, correct? Exactly why "fast and easy" is never supposed to imply "risky and unpredictable" here in America.

There is, of course, a pecking order of trust that further aids Americans in making choices when it comes to their actions. A January, 2020 article published in "MarketWatch" ("Americans trust Amazon and Google more than the police or the government") takes note of the most trusted brands, public figures and institutions in the US. In the study that was done and referred to in the article, subjects were asked to consider entities such as teachers, law enforcement officers, doctors, public figures and celebrities. Included was the question of whether the subjects trusted information from health and weather advisories or scientific studies.

Score one for the family doc. Fifty percent of subjects – the greatest share – trusted their family doctor to do the right thing. The military was listed next at 44%. Somehow Hollywood scored only a 4% share, with Wall Street at 5%, the US government at 7%, capitalism at 14% and religious leaders at 15%. In between, Amazon took 39% and Google 38%, followed by extreme weather warnings, teachers, the police, scientific studies, and health warnings or advisories. Tom Hanks and Oprah also beat out the president and Warren Buffett.

So, what does this have to do with optimum medical care? On the surface, I suppose it means that people trust their family doctor more than Tom Hanks or Wall Street to provide their medical care. That's a good thing, as trust is an extremely important part of the doctor-patient relationship. Given that good medical care can mean the difference between life and death, it's indispensable to have formed relationships with trusted clinicians in the event those situations should ever present.

What about your regular medical care for less emergent, but still urgent, situations? We all know that it's time to go straight to the emergency room if the bungee cord at Jim and Bob's broke and you dropped thirty feet directly onto cement. What if you have a cough? What if your eye is red and your lashes were stuck shut when you woke up this morning? What if you have abdominal pain – off and on? Not severe, yet not going away?

In an ideal world, you would own your own hospital and have instant access to an ophthalmologist for your eye problem, a pulmonologist for your cough, and a surgeon to evaluate your abdominal pain. For the rest of us, there is a sweet spot somewhere between having no access to care, and indeed owning your own hospital. For you economists out there, we'll call it the "affordability spot" on the Laffer Curve of medicine – the place where you get your care; care that you would like to believe is optimum.

At its heart, optimum care means care where the diagnosis is correct, the treatment is correct, and both are done in a timely manner – with the care being accessible and affordable. The latter means nothing if either of the former is incorrect. Which means that Tom Hanks should avoid practicing medicine and stick to playing astronauts and airline pilots. Which also means that care that is done in a timely, accessible and affordable manner is useless, and potentially dangerous, if the diagnosis and/or treatment are incorrect.

This, of course, begs the obvious question. How do you know that the diagnosis is correct and/or the treatment is correct once you have engaged the medical system? Answer: you don't; at least not until you get better, or until the medicine you are taking makes your eyelashes fall out. Why, then, would you engage the medical system at all, given that lack of certainty? Answer: two reasons, and they both relate to a risk/benefit ratio. First, you wouldn't engage the medical system at all if you felt that there was more risk than potential benefit in doing so. (On a more subconscious basis, the same type of reasoning is behind your choice to get up each morning and take the risk of driving to work.) Indeed, many individuals do take their chances and choose to not engage Western medicine at all. They are not convinced that the risk is worth the potential benefit.

The second reason you allow yourself to engage the system is that you've developed enough trust in

Western medicine or in your "provider" (I hate that word) of choice. (To me, the word "provider" conjures up more of an image of the world's oldest profession than it does of a medical clinician.) In any case, your level of trust allows you to engage a system where potential risks are always present in its use – more risks than eating the roadside shrimp, and risks as serious as the bungee cord rupturing.

So, who wouldn't trust a large medical conglomerate that owns hospitals, and all sorts of shiny new multiple-story buildings, when they advertise their telemedicine services with the following: "Get the same great care as an office visit?" Certainly, their doctors buy in completely to the provision of urgent care by telemedicine for just about any condition imaginable, right? Certainly, their doctors were consulted as to how the telemedicine process would be set up, how it would work, and – most importantly – what conditions as presented by patients would be routed through for a telemedicine visit, right? Certainly their doctors were trained in the intricacies of providing care by telemedicine, more so than just the nuts and bolts of getting connected with their patients and figuring out how to have them stick their iPhones down their throats to try to get a peek at their tonsils, right? Certainly, in a rush to capitalize on the new age of telemedicine, a large medical conglomerate would not attempt to direct as many patients as possible toward video visits – even if they already had presented at a clinic to be seen for a face-to-face visit, right? Certainly…Certainly.

Likewise, who wouldn't trust a slick online medical "provider" (here the term is more appropriate) with a picture of a handsome young clinician on the first page? Said clinician notes how easy it is to book an online appointment and that "we can treat (almost) anything" simply through a visit on your phone. The subsequent list is almost endless: "prescriptions, antibiotics, diabetes, refills, birth control, gout, hypertension, PrEP, pneumonia, hypothyroidism, lipid regulators, IBS, asthma, depression, ear infection, acne, anxiety, STDs, sinus infection, erectile dysfunction, cough, flu, UTI… and almost anything else!" Why stop there? Surely, the home appendix removal kit is right around the corner.

How about this bit of telemedicine advertising: "The last thing you want to do is trek across town to see a doctor." Perhaps, then, we should add a line to Jim and Bob's sign that would read: "The last thing you want to do is drive another two miles up the road to where the bungee jumping is safety monitored."

By now it should be obvious to patients that Western medicine has, in fact, been lying to everyone for decades – hell, for centuries. No one ever really needed to be examined in person by a doctor. It just took until now, when technology would allow, for us to admit that an interaction on a screen is, in fact, superior to an interaction in person.

Okay. Now that I've had time to rant, let me back up the train again. As I noted in the introduction to this book, telemedicine has a definite place in the current delivery of medical care. In fact, in some instances, and some circumstances, it is the best available modality through which to access certain kinds of care. There is no doubt that, in remote areas, or in small hospitals without immediate access to specialty care, telemedicine can be a godsend as a conduit to that specialty care. There are also certain services (such as diabetic consults or mental health visits) that, while still best delivered by face-to-face visits, can be reasonably achieved through telemedicine consults when circumstances demand. In early 2020, as we all know, circumstances regarding medical care changed drastically, and the CMS (Center for Medicare and Medicaid Services) decided that the rules previously governing the delivery of and remuneration for telemedicine services would also be changed drastically, in an effort to continue to support the provision of medical care during the Covid-19 pandemic. (More on that in Chapter Four.)

Large health care systems took notice – immediately. Certainly, their doctors bought in to the provision of urgent care by telemedicine for just about any condition imaginable. Certainly their doctors were consulted about how the telemedicine process would be set up, how it would work, and what conditions as presented by patients would be routed through for a telemedicine visit. Certainly their doctors were trained in the intricacies of providing care by telemedicine, more so than just the nuts and bolts of getting connected and instructing patients on how to swallow their iPhones down to the level of their tonsils. Certainly, the control of the narrative, and therefore the control of the delivery of medical care in the United States, is in the hands of your trusted clinician.

Don't bet on it.

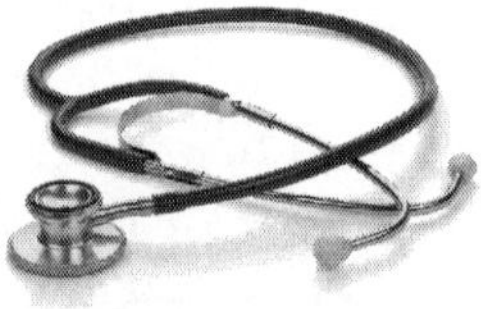

Chapter Two

Who controls the narrative, and the delivery of care?

One in every eight Americans currently works in the healthcare sector – on the face of it, an almost staggering statistic. Lots of jobs for lots of people – and therefore open to a major blow when the sector takes a hit. The healthcare sector had not been used to taking big hits – and then, 2020 arrived. In a New York Times article published May 8, 2020, Margo Singer-Kats notes: "For more than half a century, in good economic times and bad, healthcare jobs in the United States just kept increasing. Economists and health analysts thought of them as nearly recession proof: a buffer against the business cycle. But like so many other patterns, the coronavirus pandemic has broken this relationship. With the virus and its fallout deterring Americans from using the health system, job losses started in March and accelerated to 1.4 million last month."

As an example of the hit that healthcare took in early 2020, it was reported that the U.S. GDP took a 4.8% drop in the first quarter. Of that 4.8%, 2.3% was attributed to losses in the healthcare sector, with some early estimates of over 50% revenue drops in group practices. I present this information as evidence that, at the dawn of the "new age of telemedicine" – early 2020 – the healthcare sector in the United States was falling into deep financial doo-doo. It is understandable, based on this reality, that the healthcare sector would do what it felt was necessary to remain financially solvent. The gift horse that trotted their way – courtesy of the CMS – was one that was freshly tamed. The gift horse was not at all like its telemedicine predecessor, a wild pony that could not be ridden at all in the way that health plans had desired. Not that health plans/healthcare conglomerates hadn't tried to ride the wild pony before. They had, but not with the success that the gift horse, already broken by the CMS, could potentially provide. (More details in Chapter Four.)

With the potential uses of telemedicine now being wide open – and reimbursements changed by CMS to match those of a regular office visit – significantly increasing telemedicine services could help provide a way out of the financial morass that Covid-19 had created. An idea whose time had come: a way to generate similar reimbursements with no office space and very little reception or nursing personnel. And – better yet – patients needing care that were willing to avoid the potential exposures that might come with an in-person office visit. Sounds like a win-win-win. It is, as long as you control the narrative, and your narrative reads "Get the same great care as an office visit."

Why should this matter to patients? It should matter to patients because, in order to make informed decisions, patients need to know who really controls the delivery of their medical care. In order to make those decisions, they need to be aware of the factors that might influence the treatments they receive. Otherwise, it just goes like this: 1) Bill's employer pays his healthcare premium (around 55% of the U.S. population receives health insurance paid for by their employer – with around 67% of the total population carrying private insurance and around 34% receiving public coverage); 2) Bill's plan directs him to clinics that are covered under his plan. Given our previous stat about the decline of independent medical practices in the United States – 3) Bill is most likely to end up getting care at a clinic that is run by a corporate entity. And this is an issue, because…?

It is an issue because corporations are driven by profit. "So what" you say, "aren't independent practice physicians also driven by profit?" Indeed, they are, as are most ventures where people are working to make a living. However, given the fiduciary responsibility of corporations to their shareholders and stakeholders, when the excrement hits the turbine, the need to create profit will always rise to the top of the sludge that is left over. Physicians, on their own, have an oath of responsibility that goes first to their patients, and later to profit.

Witness (in a 10/18/2020 St. Paul Pioneer Press article) the thought process of the head of one of the largest health care systems in the upper Midwest out-and-out telling primary physicians and their patients how their care should be handled: "Last year, Fairview CEO James Hereford – who joined the organization in 2016 – signaled an interest in cutting costs, centralizing healthcare and moving toward virtual visits. 'Basically half the care we provide in primary care doesn't need or require a physical visit,' said Hereford, in a March 2019 interview with the Pioneer Press. 'So, how do we provide care that allows you to pick up the phone, to do a video chat, to be able to do a secure message back and forth to get your needs met?'"

Should we take a little vote here? How many believe that Mr. Hereford (educational background in math) unequivocally has quality patient care at the head of his list, and how many believe that the need to create profit is rising to the top of the sludge? We're voting for a single choice here because quality of care eventually gets impacted by increasing levels of "cost containment" (read: "increasing profits"). As you are deciding which voting lever to pull, keep in mind that what is generally fed to you from corporate-run medical care here in the land of OZ is generated from quite a curtain – er, contingent – of PR people, whose number one job is to extoll the virtues of the health plan wizard. Occasionally, as above, we get a peek behind the curtain.

If you still haven't voted, perhaps this will help. Let's examine some key issues related to the "corporatization" of medicine by looking back at history, and by examining current practicing physician viewpoints.

Concern about corporations and their possible influence on the practice of medicine was an issue way back in 1847, when the American Medical Association first conceived the essentials of the legal entity now known as the Corporate Practice Of Medicine Doctrine. The idea then was to protect the public, but also to protect doctors themselves, and their profession. The AMA "sought to establish the autonomy of medical doctors as independent decision-makers who cared for nothing but the scientific treatment of patients." Since then, the Corporate Practice Of Medicine Doctrine continues to be redefined through state law. A current overview that follows is provided by the AMA:

"The corporate practice of medicine doctrine prohibits corporations from practicing medicine or employing a physician to provide professional medical services. This doctrine arises from state medical practice acts and is based on a number of policy concerns, such as (1) allowing corporations to practice medicine or employ physicians will result in commercialization of the practice of medicine, (2) a corporation's obligation to its shareholders may not align with a physician's obligation to his patients, and (3) employment of a physician by a corporation may interfere with the physician's independent medical judgment. While most states prohibit the corporate practice of medicine, almost every state has brought exceptions, such as for professional corporations and employment of physicians.

While there are "rules" as outlined by states to prohibit corporations from practicing medicine, complex and insidious intrusions into that realm continue to plague clinical care.

Doctor Gene Uzawa Dorio, a practicing internal medicine physician, offers up an interesting summary on the social media physician site KevinMD.com. "Nowadays, it is commonplace for insurance companies to deny doctor ordered care with a simple explanation: 'not covered.' Medication is changed without physician authorization, diagnostic procedures are denied, and hospitals pressure doctors to discharge patients, sometimes too early. The public must wonder why educated professionals are now marginalized in medical decision-making within their own field."

He goes on: "Protective CPM laws have been whittled away, distorted by healthcare corporations as 'archaic' and 'detrimental' to advancing patient care. They want shareholders to benefit, while the public suffers. Interference in doctor decision-making is now more profound in all aspects of medicine. Specifically, templated strategies have been crafted by hospital lobbyists and administrators to legally avoid the appearance of physician-controlled employment. Instead, they have signed contracts with doctor groups (ER on-call specialists, radiologists, pathologist, anesthesiologist, cardiologist) controlling them financially, and often influencing patient care. The corporate practice of medicine is really the corporate control of medicine. This is why doctors are marginalized in decision-making, yet the public has not grasped this reality. On the horizon, medical care will only deteriorate as these healthcare corporations further erode protective CPM laws. To what degree must the public be financially assaulted with increasing premiums, larger deductibles, non-covered medical fees, and outrageous hospital bills before they say 'enough?' And when will we realize the complex legalese and barriers placed before us when we are told: You cannot choose your doctor; you cannot go to a specialist; you cannot have a CT scan; you must change your medication; etc."

Physicians are well aware that their autonomy in the practice of medicine has been, and continues to be, steadily eroded. The number one reason physicians point to regarding their loss of autonomy, per the journal Medical Economics, is prior authorization. Prior authorization is a complex process used by many health insurance companies as a "utilization management tool" in deciding whether certain medications or procedures or services may be covered. It is a laborious, time-consuming, frustrating process that – despite the amount of time spent – often still doesn't succeed in convincing the twenty-year-old clerk at the other end of the line that your patient's needs are crucial. It's an experience that many of us dealt with that later led us to self-prescribe primal scream therapy.

Regarding other intrusions, despite a number of good things that can be ascribed to the use of an electronic medical record, primal scream therapy has also often been a necessary response to its use. Doctor Danielle Ofri recently published an article in the New York Times, entitled "The Business of Health Care Depends on Exploiting Doctors and Nurses." She notes: "By now, corporate medicine has milked just about all the 'efficiency' it can out of the system. With mergers and streamlining, it has pushed the productivity numbers about as far as they can go. But one resource that seems endless – and free – is the professional ethic of medical staff members… By far the biggest culprit of the mushrooming workload is the electronic medical record or EMR. It has burrowed its tentacles into every aspect of the healthcare system... Primary care doctors spend nearly 2 hours typing into the EMR for every one hour of direct patient care." She further notes: "From 1975 to 2010, the number of healthcare administrators increased 3,200%. There are now roughly 10 administrators for every doctor. If we converted even half of those salary lines to additional nurses and doctors, we might have enough clinical staff members to handle the work. Health care is about taking care of patients, not paperwork."

Why so much data input into the EMR? All of this for patient care? Hardly. Types of data collected through the EMR are both quantitative and qualitative.

While the data is often used for clinical studies purposes, the CMS and healthcare organizations have their own "quality" financial and marketing interests in mind when it comes to how they believe medicine should be practiced – and now have a readily inputted (and forced) source of data to mine. "Meaningful Use," or "[EHR-MU]," was one such CMS program. It ran from 2009 through 2018 before being sent to the great acronym beyond. It was subsequently reincarnated as a part of "MIPS" – programs basically set up to input and share patient data. Physicians could potentially get "rewarded" for good behavior, and penalized if they chose not to participate. The rules set up by CMS for these programs read like the instructions for bolting together a large outdoor gazebo – written in Chinese.

Mega-corporate medicine was, of course, more than happy to use EMR data to attempt to mine the elusive gold dust that CMS had sprinkled around. To do so meant that they were more than happy to force physician compliance with "quality initiative" programs like "No one will ever get prescribed an antibiotic until they are near death, and maybe not even then" (a title unfortunately too long for its own acronym). To effectively mine that gold dust meant that corporate middle-management types had to employ constant vigilance, lest its physicians slip up and use a diagnosis like "bronchitis" to describe their patient's symptoms. Doing that, while simultaneously using their expertise to determine that their patients actually needed an antibiotic, meant that physicians would putting the corporation at risk for unsuccessful mining. Never mind that this type of pressure on physicians could affect the types of appropriate care decisions that were being made between doctors and patients.

So, corporations figured out how they could make a few extra bucks using an EMR. Rather quickly, they also figured out how they could save a few bucks using an EMR – by making their clinicians create medical records without transcription costs. This may get us a bit into the weeds, but it is an important issue to examine within the goal of understanding the reach of corporate (and government) medical America, and how that reach affects your medical care – right down to how the details of your doctor's office visit get entered into your medical chart.

Historically, starting in the 1920s, paper chart medical records were first used in the United States. These were records that were written by hand for many years until physicians began dictating their notes, which were then typed and placed in a patient's chart by transcriptionists. These notes were quite simple at first, but over time became more voluminous as the insurance industry demanded more complex documentation to justify the levels of charges that physicians were inputting. Dictations also became more complex over time as a response to medical-legal concerns.

Fast-forward to 2004, when President George W. Bush promoted the use of electronic medical records during his State of the Union address – outlining a goal that electronic health records would be available to most Americans within 10 years. That proclamation came on the heels of a report by the Institute of Medicine (IOM) in 1999, entitled "To Err is Human." The IOM more recently changed that somewhat Orwellian-sounding moniker to now be known as the "National Academy of Medicine." The "NAM" is actually a non-government, non-profit arm of the National Academy of Sciences, and the studies it does can be requested by independent or federal agencies or be specific mandates by Congress. Their report had suggested that electronic order entry systems instead of hand written orders for prescription drugs could likely decrease a number of medication errors thought responsible for some of the 98,000 deaths occurring annually as a result of overall healthcare errors. Implementation, however, proved to be slower than expected, and by 2011 physicians were being plied with Medicare incentives over the next five years in order to adopt EMRs. Arising out of these efforts was also the previously mentioned infamous "carrot and stick" program known as "meaningful use."

Back to the inputting of medical records, and as we examine how that ties to the corporate control of medicine, remember that the implied original goal of the implementation of the EMR was to improve cost and quality of care – and primarily to help reduce medical error. In fact, the EMR does help reduce certain medical errors. Without a doubt, the input of medication orders into an EMR system is much safer than the risks involved in interpreting handwritten orders for the same medications. Without a doubt, the amount of data instantly available at your fingertips in an EMR versus a paper chart is astounding. And, without a doubt, the risk of creating error in the current (and often compulsory) method of medical record charting in an EMR is also astounding.

Why the risk of error here, and why "compulsory?" I use the word compulsory because many large healthcare systems currently do not allow their clinicians the option to dictate their patient encounter notes to transcription, instead requiring them to electronically create their own notes. Why? Because transcriptions cost corporations money. Compelling clinicians to create their own notes electronically bypasses the step of having to pay someone else to transcribe a dictated Before the advent of the EMR, dictation by a clinician was the modern primary method of documenting a patient encounter. Those dictations would then be transcribed (or more recently, sent through voice recognition technology) and then entered into the medical record. There they could later be reviewed (and errors corrected, if necessary) before being signed off by the clinician. Notes Kayla Matthews (Health IT Outcomes, 12/2019 – "Why Medical Dictation Is Still Better Then Voice recognition... For Now"): "The comparison and accuracy of these two methods is crucial since the smallest error can result in injury or death. In nearly every study, speech recognition had a higher rate of error than transcription. AI voice recognition accuracy ranges from 88.9 to 96 percent, though vendors often market these products as 99% effective. Dictation and transcription, however, have a 99.6 percent accuracy rate, significantly reducing the risk of error and malpractice."

The advent of the EMR opened the opportunity for all patient encounter notes to be directly entered (electronically) into the record, which in turn, opened the window for error. To be fair – at this point – is important to note that while corporate medicine may have opened a "compulsory" window for error here, many physicians eagerly chose to save themselves documentation time by choosing to jump through it.

Those who chose to jump could have chosen a much more error-free approach than they did, rather than choosing the quicker but more error-prone world of cloned dictation (which I'll describe shortly). They could have chosen to type their notes directly into the system (though the speed at which many physicians type would make that impractical for them). They could have chosen to free-flow directly dictate into the EMR (as some do) by using an instant voice recognition technology such as Dragon. This is not altogether a bad option, though many systems do not allow such a note to be pended and then reviewed later for errors, but instead require it to be rapidly reviewed and signed off before the clinician can move on. Not having time to more thoroughly review this type of note also increases the risk of uncorrected errors.

Interestingly, some physicians who obviously have chosen not to read and correct their voice recognition notes have also decided that they are somehow "safe" by adding the following caveat at the end of those notes: "Dictation was performed using voice recognition software. There may be errors in dictation, secondary to voice recognition anomalies." Seeing these always makes me shake my head. Your "caveat" has just served up your head on a legal platter, as well as told the next clinician that they may not be able to completely trust your note.

A safer alternative to this free flow "front-end dictation" is "back-end dictation," where clinicians free flow dictate and speech recognition technology later generates a text. The completed text is available when the clinician has time for a more thorough review of the note before signing off.

The error problem with electronically created patient encounter notes, though, is not so much with these approaches as it is with a process used to help create notes known as "cloning." "Cloned documentation," as defined by CMS, is "multiple entries in a patient's health record that are exactly alike or similar to other entries in the same patient's health record or another patient's health record." How did this process come about? The day it became possible to electronically enter information into a patient's record to create a clinical encounter note was the day the concept of cloning was born. It didn't take some clinicians long to realize that their task of creating clinical encounter notes could be significantly shortened by copying previous information from their patient's (or other) records into their patient's current note – or by creating templated history and exam information they could use over and over in creating notes. It's not hard to see how the "garbage in, garbage out" concept ends up playing out here.

When you drop in a templated physical exam note in a medical chart that states: "The patient is noted to have a small, smooth, non-tender and non-nodular prostate," and the chart belongs to a 13-year-old female (as has happened) it may just slightly decrease the credibility of the rest of your note. At least, if these notes were carefully read before being signed off, these types of errors could be corrected. A JAMA Network article from July 1, 2018, on the "Analysis of Errors in Dictated Clinical Documents Assisted by Speech Recognition Software and Professional Transcriptionists," underscores the issue: "An observed error rate of more than 7% in speech recognition generated clinical documents demonstrates the importance of manual editing and review."

So, what's the big deal? Everyone is aware that a 13-year-old biological female does not have a prostate. The big deal is that "efficiency tools" may save clinicians time, but they may also create medical record information that is inaccurate, adds to fraud risk for billing, and increases the risk of liability. The big deal for patients is that inaccurate medical information can lead to medical errors. The big deal for clinicians is the risk of creating those medical errors, and of creating medical records where the use of cloning is quite obvious – especially to attorneys.

A professional medical liability organization known as the Norcal Group put out a stellar paper on June 30, 2017, entitled "Optimize Your EHR to Manage Risks: Case Studies, and Best Practices." In it they outline the types of issues that can occur with records created by efficiency tools, including: "Information that belongs to a different patient. Attestation statements from the wrong physician. Vital signs that never change. Text that is identical to entries in the physicians other patient records. Personal pronouns that switch back and forth between genders. Documentation of obviously incorrect normal examination findings (e. g., documentation of a normal cervix in a patient who has had a total hysterectomy)." The fact that medical errors – significant ones – can occur as a result of these issues is obvious.

One would think that CMS would weigh in strongly here, but the fact that they haven't taken much of a solid stand on cloning is confusing. I was surprised to learn this in the course of doing some research for a recent keynote speech I did on EMR use to a health information management convention. Perhaps the CMS "stand" on cloning is based more on their being vested in how medical services are charged rather than in a concern for medical errors. Their real interest in cloning appears to be related to coding levels for charges that seem to be increasing based on the ability now to use a few clicks in an EMR to create more detailed documentation, and therefore justify those increased charges.

The speech I gave to the health information management group was entitled "The EMR: Protecting the Patient – and Ourselves," and explored the issues related to the paper chart versus the EMR – reviewing what is good documentation and how the EMR could either help or hinder good documentation. I noted that, for the benefit of patients and clinicians alike, a good medical record should be one where its reader can quickly find and understand the assessment and treatment plan for the visit. The reader of a good medical record should also be able to easily access ancillary data such as lab and x-ray results, and easily find and understand the observed and historical data that support the plan from the visit.

Cloned and templated medical records easily lead to "note bloat" and an increased risk for medical errors. I noted that the CMS did not appear to have a specific policy against cloning, but that their statement on it at the time noted that "it is a problem in healthcare institutions that is not broadly addressed." CMS had further clarified their position at the time, noting: "Healthcare professionals have stated that copying and pasting notes can be appropriate and eliminate the need to create every part of a note and re-interview patients about their medical histories. However, the HHS – OIG (the U.S. Department of Health and Human Services Office of Inspector General) identifies 'illegitimate use of cut and paste record cloning' as a problem."

All fine and good – except for the fact that there was no further definition from CMS as to what "illegitimate use" actually constitutes. I noted to those in attendance that a University of California, San Francisco study of 500 clinicians over an eight-month period using an inpatient Epic EMR had found that over 80% of the notes they created were imported or copied from elsewhere, and only 18% of the text was actually entered manually. I also referenced another major study – from Methods of Information in Medicine – which showed that 84% of all notes in their investigation contained at least one documentation error, with an average of 7.8 documentation problems per patient. In that study, copying another physician's note and making changes resulted in the highest rate of error.

Corporate medicine is as aware of this data as much as anyone else. Corporate medicine should have a problem with this, but doesn't really appear to. Perhaps the bean counters have decided that this particular "cost of business" decision outweighs its attendant risks. Clinicians shouldn't be left off the hook here either, whether they profess to understand the risks or not, as they have an ethical duty to be aware of them, and to act accordingly. Last, but certainly not least, government (as a payor) should have more of a problem with this. Instead, if anything, CMS relaxed their rules regarding cloned documentation before they ushered in changes to coding for office visits beginning in January, 2021.

In an October 12, 2020 article entitled "CMS update on medical record documentation for E/M services," the author (from Codingintel.com) notes that "the OIG expressed concerns about copy/paste and over-documentation in 2014, but this did not lead to CMS standards about the practice." She added that "CMS is now allowing physicians to' review and verify' rather than re-document the history and exam," further stating that, " it would seem that CMS does not care about the issue of copying and pasting from a prior record."

As it goes clinically, the history and physical are the most important components of a patient visit, and it would seem that CMS does not care about them either. The above noted January, 2021 changes (by CMS) in coding rules for outpatient office visits were actually about office visit charges, and were supposedly designed to make it easier for physicians to determine and enter those charges. "Easier" may or may not be true, but the significant change made was that the history and physical exam part of the visit were no longer to be factored in as part of the documentation to support a visit charge. In essence, the clinically most important part of the visit note would no longer be considered regarding the value of the visit.

Was this change by CMS intended to decrease the amount of information cloned into medical records? I suspect not, and it won't likely decrease it much in those who already copy/paste create their medical records. CMS doesn't appear to care if clinicians clone – they just want to decrease any possible reimbursement benefit from doing so. Even though the stated intention of their new coding rules was to make it easier for physicians to document and enter charges, history has led most physicians to tend to look askance at any offering of "altruism" emanating from CMS.

Charge documentation under the new guidelines was switched to be based either on MDM (medical decision-making) or on the amount of time spent by the clinician for the visit. More physician activities during the visit can now be counted as "time" under the new rules, but the amount of "time" that needs to be documented to justify most levels of charges has also been markedly increased. So, while some chart "note bloat" may go away, others forms of note bloat will need to be created in order for physicians to get paid. Altruism on the part of CMS? Looks more like another shot at limiting reimbursements without any concern for the issues created by medical record cloning. Who ends up being at the most risk as a result of medical record cloning? Patients, of course. Patients are the ones who run the biggest risk from adverse outcomes due to medical errors. Perhaps next time you are in for an office visit, you ought to ask your doctor about how she or he creates your medical records?

One of the other burgeoning areas of EMR use that also affects both physicians and patients is what is referred to as computerized clinical decision support systems or CDSS. These are software programs that are designed (ostensibly) to be an aid to physicians in clinical decision-making. The Institute of Medicine helped promote these after the American Recovery and Reinvestment Act of 2009 had advocated further endorsement of health information technology.

CDSS programs are designed with a number of functions, with the only truly useful one I've seen as a physician being the patient safety function, which will elicit warnings on drug-to-drug interactions (even though at times these are wrong) as well as medication allergies. As far as the clinical management and diagnosis support functions of CDSS, I will stick to first trusting my brain. "Diagnosis support" for imaging in some cases now includes a list of clinical questions designed to "suggest" to the clinician whether or not their imaging order is appropriate in the workup of the patient. I will presume that my patient from a couple of months ago is happy that he had his inflamed appendix removed after I disregarded the CDSS suggestion that my order of a CT scan of his abdomen was not warranted. This is just one of many instances where experienced physicians will decide to bypass the "suggestion" and await the surely soon to come slap on the hand (financial or otherwise) for not bowing to their EMR.

Unfortunately, the less than subtle coercion to comply with corporate medical mandates does not stop there. Enter the wonderful world of rating systems. You have undoubtedly used one form of rating system or another to avoid that crappy plate of pasta we mentioned earlier. Your use of the rating system may have been helpful, or perhaps not. Why? Because the value of the information you are relying on depends almost exclusively on the value of the information that was entered into the system in the first place – again, the old "garbage in, garbage out" axiom. Perhaps you thought that the moo goo gai pan you devoured at the Orange Dragon Restaurant last night was the best meal you had ever eaten. You were disappointed that the restaurant got only two stars for that dish on your restaurant rating system, until closer inspection revealed a small sample size – three total raters, two of whom unfortunately received food not warm enough to their liking. While rating systems can assist and influence consumers in a number of arenas, flaws in the systems are rampant – again, not a huge issue when you get a crappy plate of pasta, but indeed a huge issue when it comes to your health care.

Jessie Zheng, and Janice Coffin, D.O., explain the STAR rating system for physicians in a March 18, 2020 article in Medical Economics, entitled "Improving quality and increasing star ratings." They note: "Medicare and Medicaid make up 38% of medical payments in the United States. Whether working in a private practice or a health network, a large number of patients will be receiving benefits from these programs run through the Centers for Medicare and Medicaid services (CMS). By accepting payments through federal payers and contracted Medicare Advantage (MA) plans, physicians are held to the quality standards set by CMS and the National Center for Quality Assurance (NHQA). These standards were established in 1991 and are updated yearly to reflect changes in value-based care goals and standard of care guidelines. With an increasing focus on value-based care, physicians can expect a larger focus on these quality measures. The Healthcare Effectiveness Data Information Set (HEDIS) is divided into six domains of care." The authors go on to note that these six domains include utilization, access and availability of care, health plan descriptive information measures collected using electronic clinical data systems, effectiveness of care, and my favorite – "experience of care."

They go on: "HEDIS defines how these quality measures are to be collected by payers for evaluation of both providers and insurance plans. Collection methods can include billing claims, surveys or clinical documentation from office visits or labs. Once collected, measures are tallied into a 5-Star rating for private payers using predetermined Core Quality Measures stratified for different medical specialties. As these ratings are tied to CMS reimbursement bonuses, there are incentives at multiple levels to reach either the 4- or 5-star rating tiers. Many insurance companies have their own programs designed to help providers meet these measures through education, tools, and bonuses. Pay-for-performance programs include flat fee bonuses for each patient meeting a measure or a percentage bonus for a practice if it meets a certain rating threshold."

Primary care doctors know that measures that are particularly important to HEDIS include preventative screening, such as breast cancer screening and colon cancer screening, as well as diabetes treatment and screening and medication adherence. So, your doctor needs to make sure that he or she discusses these issues thoroughly with you in order for you to understand their importance, and it ends there – correct? Not exactly, as most patients have discovered when telling their primary care doctors that they do not wish to have certain screening procedures or take certain medications. Would your insurance company really push your doctor to push you into "compliance?" Zheng and Coffin note: "A representative from United Healthcare Regional Operations says a common misconception is that documenting non-adherence can help close care gaps such as refusal to take medication or perform screening tests. Only a few specific exclusions, such as intolerance to the listed drugs or end-stage renal disease are usually accepted."

In other words, if you as a physician don't force compliance, it's counted against you – financially, and in your ratings – ratings viewable on the Physician Compare website. With this in mind, I'm not surprised that I've lost count of the number of patients that have come to me in urgent care over the last eighteen years to take care of issues commonly handled by their primary care physician. When I ask why they aren't seeing their primary physician instead, they are usually quite forthcoming in telling me that they got tired of trying to be forced into doing something they didn't want to do. "They said they wouldn't refill my blood pressure medicines unless I let them put a three-foot rubber tube up my butt," a rather spry elderly lady told me one day. "So, here I am."

Is working with physicians in an attempt to improve the quality of care provided in medical encounters a bad thing? Obviously, not. The important operative words to keep in mind in that sentence, however, are "working with." Is it problematic, by various types of coercion, to attempt to control physicians to meet corporate designed endpoints? Hell, yes. Do you really want your doctor to be bullied into providing care that is geared toward maintaining a stellar corporate star rating?

Primary care doctor Lisa Ravindra opines in an article in The Hill ("Give it 5 stars: How doctor ratings affect your health care. Nov.30, 2020): "A 2018 study in JAMA reported that telemedicine patients who received an antibiotic for a respiratory tract infection (e.g. a "cold") gave high ratings. This is concerning since respiratory tract infections are usually viral and rarely warrant antibiotic use, which can lead to dangerous outcomes for patients."

She goes on: "To be sure, checks and balances on physicians are undoubtedly important. While physicians take an oath to do no harm, no industry is free from bad actors… Monitoring by state medical boards and hospital quality assurance committees are traditional ways to ensure patient safety. When seeking medical care, patients can view online reviews with the understanding that they can be flawed, biased and subjective. Patients deserve the best healthcare possible, and need to understand good ratings do not always lead to good doctors. Save the stars for the restaurants, not the physicians."

It is important to remember here that your physician's health plan employer also has access to ratings data for physicians that can be used for purposes of compensation, and to determine the advisability of continued employment. Physicians are well aware of this .

As to what primarily motivates so many other enterprises, Marion Mass accurately notes: "follow the money." In an article in MedPage Today, "American Healthcare: Increasingly Corporate and Rapacious," Dr. Mass eloquently outlines how corporations, with large administrative and managerial overheads, "suck in vast amounts of money, and they spend part of that money making sure the rules of the road in American healthcare favor them, not the patient." She points out the largest corporate entities at fault – especially large pharmacies, pharmacy benefit managers, and consolidated hospitals. She fortunately also offers some initiatives worth supporting in order to help minimize the fallout, which we will further discuss in Chapter Seven.

I will presume by now that you have gotten the hint that your primary care or urgent care doctor likely doesn't have the control over your medical care that you may have thought he or she did. I could go on and on with more examples (but that would just prove what my wife has said about me all along).

Back to why this should matter to patients. That should be obvious by now – and perhaps even more obvious in the wake of the coronavirus pandemic. Let's invoke a quote attributed to Doctor Emanuel's brother Rahm: "You never want a serious crisis to go to waste. And what I mean by that [is], it's an opportunity to do things that you think you could not before."

Surely you would not be offered, or pushed toward, a telemedicine visit for your condition if it was not really appropriate for telemedicine.

Don't bet on it.

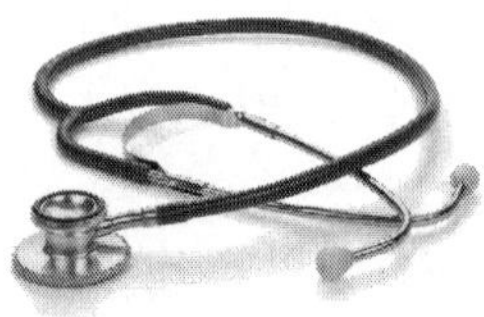

Chapter Three Enter Technology

"Technology is a useful servant but a dangerous master." – Christian Louis Lange, Historian

Technological advances seem to be coming toward us today in an exponential fashion. Concerns about technological wonders versus pitfalls, however, have been with us for centuries. Social scientists like to consider Mary Shelley an early in-the-trenches alarmist, with her tale of a created monster that helped point out the ugly downside of unregulated technology in the early age of the Industrial Revolution.

As today's world becomes further blessed with (as well as dependent on) technology, it behooves us to continue to examine its impact on multiple facets of our lives. Current literature is replete with glowing testimonials to the wonders that technology can deliver, as well as lists of caveats that might make us second-guess how fast we accept technological advances that nibble at society's edges until they produce a new norm. Maybe I'm sensitive because I used to worry as a kid that one day someone in a lab would inadvertently concoct the "universal" solvent – and, of course, would have nothing to store it in. I was simultaneously comforted back then by the fact that, for six million dollars, my body could be completely rebuilt. (In today's dollars, I think that sum might still cover Steve Austin's bionic ear.) Thank God there are worse things to worry about today

– like how to get your hands on the latest piece of technological advancement.

The "all tech is good" and "more tech is always better" crowd is, of course, ready to stand in line in the rain without food, drink, or bathroom breaks for at least a week to replace their ancient eleven-month-old iPhone with the newest iteration that promises a camera that can record slow speed underwater video. On the other end, the "I'm an old fud that still drives a '68 Buick and hasn't seen a movie since 'Mary Poppins'" crowd is still probably trying to find a battery charger to juice up the old Motorola "brick" phone they bought in 1987.

It should be fairly obvious that in the case of cell phones, as in many other areas of tech advancement, the lines of adoption are often – but not always – drawn along the lines of age. Somewhere in between the "early adopters" (about 14%) and the "laggards" (about 16%), sit most of us. And so it is with doctors. Some of us are early adopters, and hopefully none of us are still answering calls on the old Motorola brick (in some cases, only because the damn thing just doesn't work anymore). A good case can often be made for sitting on either end of the spectrum.

The thalidomide scare of the late 1950s and early 1960s is often referred to by doctors who tend more toward the laggard end of the scale as they point to the dangers of early adoption of technology. In that case, thalidomide was a drug prescribed to treat morning sickness in pregnancy that unfortunately led to serious birth defects and death in thousands of children before it was removed from the market in 1961.

The fen-phen debacle of the 1990s may also be a reference point raised by later adopters. I personally do not consider myself to be a late adopter, but I know that I also avoid being a very early adopter of new medical technology, especially when that technology may be useful in treating medical conditions that are important, but not necessarily life-threatening.

Such was the case with fen-phen. The drug combination fenfluramine/phentermine – a.k.a. fen/phen – was a pharmacological treatment for obesity that combined two anorectic drugs. Fenfluramine by itself had been around since the 1970s, but when it was combined with phentermine in the 1990s, its use as a weight-loss combination drug really took off. My initial concerns about the drug were based, as much as anything, on evidence that – although the drug seemed to help early on with weight loss – the maintenance of long-term weight loss was another story. Why take any potential risks with a newer drug combination when the long-term benefits did not appear to be solid?

I distinctly remember a number of patients leaving me and my practice when I refused to prescribe the drug based on the above reasoning, and on some other concerns. I also distinctly remember that in 1997 (after the FDA pulled the drug from the market), a number of those same patients came back to me and asked me to order echocardiograms to rule out heart valve damage that was being attributed to the same drug – which they had gotten elsewhere.

Decisions for use or non-use of new technology by physicians – whether it be imaging, drugs, procedures, or other modalities – are complex ones. They involve, but are not limited to: considerations of the background of the physician; the physician's previous experience with the use of technology in general; the physician's training in the use of this technology in specific; the medical history of the patient to which the technology is being applied; the specific medical problem to which the technology is being applied; cost of the technology; potential risks and benefits of the technology; reliability of the technology; other potential options for diagnosis or treatment; ready availability of the technology; the background of the patient; the patient's previous experience with technology; and the patient's (as well as the physician's) trust regarding the specific new technology itself. That's quite a list! (Consider also: tech comfort and adaptability on the basis of age of the patient considered. Would our patient George have been comfortable showing his telemedicine doctor the site of his pain?)

Note that this list outlines considerations between only two parties – the patient and the physician. That's because, when the rubber meets the road, the only two parties whose views should really count in making these decisions are the patient and the physician.

Duties from the patient side of the equation in making these decisions include being forthright and honest about all of the above issues, asking appropriate questions to become well-informed, and following through on agreed-upon behaviors necessary to ensure the best possible outcomes.

Duties from the physician side of the equation include explaining in detail the risks and benefits associated with the use of the technology, alternatives to the use of the technology, expected potential outcomes of the use of the technology, cost of the technology (if that's a concern), and an outline of the patient's behavior necessary to ensure the best possible outcomes.

Sounds a bit complex. It is. Sometimes the entire procedure is fairly straightforward, and sometimes – depending on the complexity of the technology – it is quite time-consuming. What it should never be is a situation where the technology – specifically of concern here, telemedicine – is dumped on both parties without the above issues being addressed.

When that happens, the situation is not safe for either patient or doctor. The really important question for you as a patient then becomes: When you need to engage a doctor, which one are you going to get? The one who is willing to risk her star rating and stand up to her duties as described above? Or, a "corporate-compliant" one who also happens to be an early adopter and prefers – since the technology has been presented and therefore is expected to be used – that it is indeed put to use immediately and in all cases, without further preparation, as presented by the corporation?

In the above list of considerations for the use of new technology, reliability stands out as a consideration that should be on the top of every physicians list. Did our corporate-compliant, early adopter take reliability into consideration, or instead forge ahead with home telemedicine connections such as Zoom once telemedicine visits at home became reimbursed by CMS at the same rate as in-person office visits?

Kate Murphy is the author of "You're Not Listening: What You're Missing and Why It Matters." She makes important points about technology such as Zoom in a recent New York Times article entitled "Why Zoom Is Terrible," subtitled: "There's a reason video apps make you feel awkward and unfulfilled." She explains: "... there are reasons to be wary of the technology, beyond the widely reported security and privacy concerns. Psychologists, computer scientists and neuroscientists say the distortions and delays inherent in video communication can end up making you feel isolated, anxious and disconnected (or more than you were already). You might be better off just talking on the phone. The problem is that the way the video images are digitally encoded and decoded, altered and adjusted, patched and synthesized introduces all kinds of artifacts: blocking, freezing, blurring, jerkiness and out-of-sync audio. These disruptions, some even below our conscious awareness, confound perception and scramble subtle social cues. Our brains strain to fill in the gaps and make sense of the disorder, which makes us feel vaguely disturbed, uneasy and tired without quite knowing why."

She goes on regarding concerns with video communication: "This is foremost because human beings are exquisitely sensitive to one another's facial expressions. Authentic expressions of emotion are an intricate array of minute muscle contractions, particularly around the eyes and mouth, often subconsciously perceived, and essential to our understanding of one another. But those telling twitches all but disappear on pixelated video or, worse, are frozen, smoothed over or delayed to preserve bandwidth."

Practicing medicine as long as I have, I can tell you without a doubt that, even during face-to-face office visits, extracting pertinent information from patients in order to make sound medical decisions isn't always easy. I don't expect it to be. I also don't expect – or want – another layer of fuzziness (in this case, virtual fuzziness) to get in the way, especially when dealing with vague symptoms. In the office, as much as patients seem to dislike it, repeating their complaints a couple of times along the way before they get back to see the doctor often actually helps define complaints that started out fuzzy.

Speaking of "fuzzy," is also important to take note of the potential tech barriers to telehealth in our rural areas – primarily in regard to the issue of limited high-speed Internet access. Recent studies have indicated that around two thirds of rural and tribal areas actually have access to FCC minimum benchmark high-speed broadband. Less people in these areas also own smart phones as compared to those in urban areas, so reliance on telemedicine as an alternative source of care is not guaranteed in these areas.

As to actual clinical encounters, some things in the office are fairly straightforward, and some things on telemedicine could also be fairly straightforward, such as discussing a record of blood sugars, or the response to an increased dose of Prozac. However, things in medicine that might initially seem straightforward often turn out to be anything but straightforward. Not every red mattering eye is pinkeye, and not every cough is just a cold. Quite the contrary. No matter how "common" something may appear, the worst thing doctors can do is to be led down the "primrose path" toward the likely without considering the alternatives. (Another good reason why presenting your symptoms to Doctor Google and being told that you "may have 'Captain Morgan Disease' and need a serum porcelain test," is not the best option to pursue.) Desiring better outcomes, there are those who argue that improved "home monitoring technology" in telemedicine may be the answer to increasing its effectiveness. Unfortunately, as much as we might seek to simplify it with technology, the practice of medicine remains a complex process.

Doctors use a process called "differential diagnosis" with almost every medical condition they see, because it is often necessary to differentiate between a number of different conditions which may share similar symptoms or signs. The differential diagnosis for cough is vast (look it up sometime), even after you break it down into adult cough versus pediatric cough, dry cough versus wet cough, cough with shortness of breath or not, cough with fever or not, acute cough versus chronic cough, etc., etc., etc. Of course, we now have "differential diagnosis generators" which are supposed to aid physicians in arriving at the proper diagnosis for their patients. Another tool – which is okay, as long as it remains a tool and doesn't become relied upon as the final say by tech-reliant clinicians. Another patient of mine with abdominal pain from a couple of months back, sent by me to the ER for surgical consultation (and eventual inflamed appendix removal), was fortunate that I didn't rely solely on his CT scan results. The report had noted: "no evidence of appendicitis." As noted at the beginning of this chapter, "Technology is a useful servant but a dangerous master."

The technology issue also needs to be examined from the standpoint of the education of today's medical students – those responsible for your future care. I recently sat down with my former medical school dean, "Distinguished University Teaching Professor," and director of a med school Family Medicine Preceptorship Program, Dr. Jim Boulger. We discussed a number of issues related to technology and education. I also later participated in a Zoom (of course!) session where he and number of young physicians on the panel discussed the impact of telemedicine on Minnesota's medical workforce, medical education, and delivery of medical care.

Foremost in our initial discussions (before the Zoom session) was the question of whether we are training our new physicians to be more and more tech reliant. I can say from my personal interactions with medical students that the answer to that question is definitely "yes." Of course, as more technology becomes available, more of it will be employed, and students will take notice. But, what of the importance of the physical exam, and of the in-person interaction? We both agreed that medical education knows that the physical exam is important or there wouldn't continue to be so much emphasis placed on it. The real concern is whether those currently in training will remain cognizant of its importance.

Doctor Jalal Baig is an oncologist and writer who practices in Chicago. He opines about the dangers inherent in pushing aside the physical exam in his Dec. 21, 2020 article on the NBC News website entitled: "Covid infection makes in-person doctor exams dangerous. But patients are more than data points."

He notes: "Though it's tempting to think that the physical exam is an outdated practice that was best suited for medicine's embryonic days, the data suggest otherwise. For example, take this 2015 study published in the American Journal of Medicine, which looked at 208 cases of oversights in physical exams. It found that 63% of oversights could've been prevented merely by performing the physical examination. In addition, the shortcomings led to wrong or delayed diagnoses in 76%

of cases." He adds, "Crucially, a 2016 study published in Current Oncology concluded that mammography's in absence of physical breast examinations can miss a significant number of cancers."

Unfortunately, the developing trend of decreasing reliance on the physical exam got a further push from Covid – 19. Says Doctor Baig: "This is the milieu that medical students and medical residents, who are newly initiated into medicine, will now train in. With their time already having been reduced at bedsides before the pandemic, these new pressures may degrade the already fraught interaction and push the patient further into the computer." This, on top of a 2019 JAMA Internal Medicine study he cites which found that "new internal medicine trainees, or interns, spent almost 90% of their work time away from patients."

Tough times might require that we sometimes "do what we have to do," but they don't require that we lose sight of the big picture. As Doctor Baig eloquently sums up, "By further de-emphasizing the centrality of physical contact and the doctor-patient relationship, the SARS –CoV-2 pandemic further threatens the practice. But as the use of exam techniques and medical tools becomes more perfunctory, physicians are shedding a treasured ritual that reduces medical errors and, most important, humanizes medicine."

Alas – we can't seem to come up with one of those handheld scanners that served Dr. McCoy so well on the old Star Trek TV series. Then, we could just do away with the physical exam. Until then…

We've already scratched the surface of the issue of physicians being driven into interactions with which they do not necessarily agree (to be further explored in

Chapter 4). Certain behaviors for them and for medical students – as well as for the public – get accustomed to over time as new normals get created by actions like telemedicine "exams." Tech reliance marches on with the allure of tech as glitzy, glamorous, and somehow superior to the human touch, or the human mind.

Was Mary Shelley correct in her assumption about the monster of technology? If technology was created to be used as a tool, then it is incumbent upon us to resolve to not allow it to become more powerful than its creator – or to seduce its creators into overuse. Unfortunately, tech creations do run the risk of becoming entities unto themselves. Witness the power of Google, Twitter and Facebook. Witness social immersion so deep that user's lives often get ruled and sometimes ruined. Tech has become a drug in the hands of some, and a religion in the hand of others. Drugs and religions are also useful tools, until they become abused or create dependency in their patrons.

Perhaps the real question is: Are new technologies (including medical ones) becoming so attractive that they might impede our abilities to appropriately limit their use? Obviously, in many situations, limit we must – even with an act as simple as policing the amount of screen time for three-year-olds. In medicine, the seduction of tech may be particularly enticing, as many of the advances in medicine – particularly over the last several decades – have been largely tech driven. It is easy, of course, to get drawn into the "if some is good, more is better" trap without evaluating each new advance on its own merit – and with a modicum of caution.

Regarding the aforementioned Zoom presentation

on telemedicine's impact on medical workforce, education, and healthcare delivery, it was an interesting session. There were, I thought, some appropriate insights into the use of a telemedicine platform – including the fact that such a platform will probably work best for people who "know each other," and that triage for any visits should be done locally and not through a "phone bank." Also raised were concerns from doctors who worked with the presenters about whether telemedicine care was "good enough" for their patients, and concerns about the quality of video – especially when evaluating conditions like rashes.

What troubled me, however, was that the majority of the discussion from the physician side of the equation related more to figuring out how to adopt telemedicine into their practice than it did to examining care concerns regarding the actual use of the technology. There appeared to be an acceptance of the fact that if your healthcare "system" told you that you would practice telemedicine, you would just do it. In particular, there was a reference to having to do a "mandated day in telemedicine" and there was no discussion, other than from Dr. Boulger, about how to react to that. His response to the idea of a mandate: "You should tell them: I'll do what's appropriate for my patients."

He went on to note that it's no great surprise that the quick adaption of telemedicine suddenly was palatable when reimbursements were increased. He also expressed his concerns about telemedicine's effect on education and the concept of "caring." One of his major concerns has been that family physicians have lost contact with each other over time, as things like traditional hospital staff meetings and staff get-togethers have been abandoned with family physicians increasingly shunning work in the hospital. This, he feels, further whittles away at Family Medicine as a profession in general. As he often notes, "Family Practice is only as strong as family docs are together."

This is a critical issue for family doctors, who are the backbone of primary care. With the ever increasing cost saving push toward nurse practitioners and physician's assistants (NPs and PAs), family medicine already faces enough of an uphill battle without a further devaluation of physician skills in favor of technology. Physicians themselves must also be careful not to devalue their worth by emphasizing lifestyle, reduced hours, and "no call" positions over being available for the patients who count on them. I honestly never thought the day would come when I would hear a primary care physician make a statement (in this case, regarding telemedicine) like, "I know it's not the best care, but I can do it from home, and…"

This brings up an important area of discussion about medical clinicians in general – and it's way past time to clear the air on this one. The issue is clinician experience. There is a seat at the table and an appropriate role for all the types of clinicians that practice medicine. Primary care physicians these days, however, stand at risk of losing their seat as corporate medicine pushes toward turning primary and urgent care practice over to NPs, PAs, and technology. Physician devaluing behavior only speeds up this process. So what, you might say, what's the problem? The problem is: I wouldn't trust the care of a neurosurgeon in a high-level urgent care, and I wouldn't trust the care of an inexperienced PA or NP there, either – nor would I trust any other doctor who isn't trained for the job. As a patient, neither should you. The issue here isn't PAs and NPs specifically, it's acute care experience, and corporate medicine isn't putting a priority on the safety of your visit if they choose to hire clinicians of any kind that don't have appropriate experience.

I have worked with NPs and PAs that were absolutely stellar practitioners of higher-level acute care medicine – and they were all experienced clinicians – clinicians who knew better than to make their first job a job where they were in way over their head. It is a huge mistake (as is being done in some quarters) to take the risk of placing fresh PA and NP graduates immediately into high-level urgent care clinics and expecting physicians (while seeing their own patients) to also help guide those fresh grads through their contacts with chest pain, shortness of breath, abdominal pain, head injuries, etc. In busy high-level acute care clinics, despite anyone's best intentions, that guidance doesn't always take place.

The risks here are first and foremost to the patient, but also to the clinician and to their physician mentor(s). On the other hand, I guess it does save corporations money… and, what the hell – who really needs appropriate experience anyway? An Ob-Gyn on board your flight from New York to Iceland could probably help handle your chest pains, right? I suppose you could sit down together and time them until they were 5 minutes apart…

Statements of fact regarding clinical experience: Physician training requires 4 years of college plus 4 years of medical school – the last 2 years of which are supervised medical rotations. After this comes minimally an additional 3 years of medical residency – again, with supervised rotations in a medical specialty.

Total time – at least 11 years. PA training requires 4 years of college plus 2 years of PA school, with that six years compressed into 5 years in some programs. NP programs require a bachelor's degree (usually 4 years) in nursing, plus 2 to 4 more years for the NP, so about 6-7 years total on average. The total hours for physician training are estimated at 20,700 to 21,700 versus 2,800 to 5,300 for NPs.

The point here is that primary care physician training programs put docs through the paces long enough that those who are comfortable doing acute care medicine have already had appropriate experience in high-end acute care by the time they graduate. (In fairness, it should be noted that many NPs also have the advantage of a significant amount of nursing experience before pursuing the NP, which does serve them well. Many a medical intern will attest to having a great nurse help bail their ass out during their training days. Twenty-some states currently allow nurse practitioners to practice independent of physician supervision.)

The goal here is not to get into some sort of pissing match about training, as the above are just statements of fact regarding training programs. All mentioned clinicians get a seat at the table. The goal here is to point out that experience matters, and in the not so distant past, doctors in medical groups got together and evaluated the colleagues they were hiring to work with them – to make sure that the skill set and experience of the applicant matched the job at hand. Corporations that choose to hire fresh, inexperienced PA/NP grads for higher-end acute care positions now often make that choice on their own, and patients need to be aware of this as they seek care. Any good doctor will tell you that extensive medical training is as much about teaching you what you need to know, as it is about teaching you what you don't know, and, when you need to ask for help.

Despite the stupidity of it all, the training "pissing match" discussion does indeed occur amongst clinicians. So, I'm here to referee. If you – doctor, PA, NP, or any other clinician – take umbrage at the experience issue described here, or if you can't check your ego at the door when it comes to admitting your limits and knowing when to seek help, that's a game misconduct penalty. If any of you are still busy trying to prove to everyone around you that your level of education is "just as good as that" of someone else, then you are completely (and potentially dangerously) missing the point, and that's also a game misconduct penalty. If any of you have never been in a clinical situation where you feel like your bowels (at least figuratively) might evacuate without your consent, then you've either been practicing massage therapy, or you haven't seen enough train wrecks to know when one is about to hit you. It's back to the minors for you. I will repeat that all of this applies to doctors as well as other clinicians – as not all doctors are built for, trained for, or comfortable with acute care medicine. Thank God, or we wouldn't have any dermatologists. Let's move on.

◆◆◆

New technology for diligent clinicians ends up being a fine line to walk between not wanting to miss out on its use as an early adopter (avoiding the "old fud" label) while at the same time not wanting to jump in too soon, before the potential dangers of that technology might become apparent. I worked with a wonderful old family doc during my internship whose concern for, and loyalty to, his patients was immense. I respected him greatly for that. I also used to cringe when he would literally spout out, "cat scan, bat scan, rat scan," when we ordered tests on his patients. About that time, young as I was, I began to suspect that there was about a three- or four-year window between when you started hearing "you look too young to be a doctor," and when the "old fud" suspicion began to creep in.

It really boils down to trust – a commodity getting progressively harder to establish over time with a physician in these days of corporate employee turnover, and in these days of EMR reliance that decreases eye-to-eye contact time. Kate Murphy adds further perspective here from her analysis of Zoom: "Video chats have also been shown to inhibit trust because we can't look one another in the eye. Depending on the camera angle, people may appear to be looking up or down or to the side. Viewers may then perceive them as uninterested, shifty, haughty, servile or guilty. For this reason, law scholars and criminal justice activists have questioned the fairness of remote depositions, hearings and trials." She notes that "… experts say no facial cues are better than faulty ones. The absence of visual input might even heighten people's sensitivity to what's being said. It could be why Verizon and AT&T have reported average daily increases of as much as 78% in voice-only calls since the start of the pandemic, as well as an increase in the length of these calls."

We, as physicians, however, remain under constant pressure to adapt to new technologies – and to do so quickly. It somehow seems that the ready answer to any new crisis presented to us is the sword of technology – ready to slay the dragon and any new crisis in medicine. We are also reminded that the (self-created) technology juggernaut continues to cruise along, with or without us. As writer Stewart Brand has remarked: "Once a new technology rolls over you, if you're not part of the steamroller, you're part of the road."

I've always found it interesting that those who aren't the ones applying the technology, and therefore not dealing with its sometimes backlash, are the ones who seem to speak loudest in its defense. Futurist Bartalan Mesko in "The Medical Futurist," March 3, 2020, writes: "… no matter how scary the future might seem at the moment, we cannot stop technological development; and, sooner or later we will find out that whole areas of our lives have been transformed through various digital technologies. Thus, our task at the moment is to face our fears about the future with courage; to turn to technologies with an open mind and to prepare for the changing world with as much knowledge as possible."

Thank God physicians aren't trained to "whip it out there and see what happens." While mistakes can and will happen, practicing physicians are trained to avoid them in any way possible, at any level – and that includes the risks of potential mistakes tied to the introduction of new technology. Having an "open mind" to practicing physicians doesn't equate to having immediately "open arms" when it comes to the application of medical tech advances. Why? Because, in most cases, practicing physicians aren't the ones who created the technologies. They, however, are the ones who get to apply them, and then, along with their patients, get to deal with the outcomes. I cannot in any way better describe the quandary created here than does Dr. Dhruv Khullar, in an April, 2018 article in the Washington Post regarding telemedicine: "As is often the case with technological change, our capacity to generate innovation has exceeded our capacity to understand its implications. With telemedicine, we've done what we usually do: Introduce a new treatment, technology or care model, and assume doctors will figure out how to use it."

That might be workable, presuming that doctors would have the time and the clout necessary to implement it in a safe, effective, and timely way. Again, with enough time, technology may improve to the point where Doctor McCoy's Star Trek handheld scanner does become a reality, and we might not need any doctor-patient interaction for a diagnosis.

Problem is – WE'RE NOT THERE YET! Until we get there, who is supposed to stand in the way long enough for telemedicine's use to be consistently safe, effective, and timely?

◆◆◆

Elinor Burkett is a best-selling activist author and good friend who has had her own recent experiences with telemedicine. We recently discussed those (more in the next chapter) and the issue of technology in medicine in general. She quite astutely pointed out that we as a society assume that tech will quickly solve our problems – and then recalled our experience as we came face-to-face with Covid-19 and discovered that tech wasn't rapidly going to save us. In the face of that, as its response, the CMS decided that the answer to making sure that its covered patients received timely medical care, regardless of the other issues, was to vastly expand the offering of telemedicine.

Desperate times may call for desperate measures, but did Thelma and Louise really have to drive a "66 Thunderbird over the edge of the Grand Canyon? Maybe yes, maybe no. Did I really need to refer to an old movie to help make my point? Definitely, no. Even without applying the brakes on the telemedicine T-Bird, the new age of telemedicine isn't going to drive us anywhere dangerous, correct?

Don't bet on it.

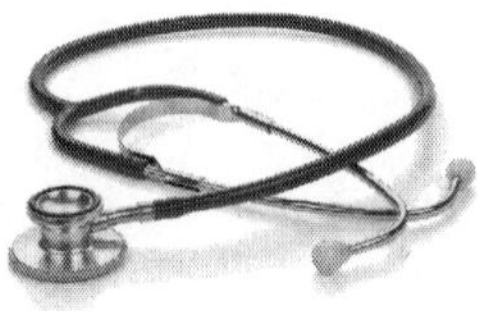

Chapter Four Telemedicine

So, we have discussed the wonders and the pitfalls of technological advances in medicine. Of all of those advances, telemedicine is now likely the most rapidly evolving. If telemedicine is indeed poised to "revolutionize" the delivery of medical care, as has been suggested, then the consumers of that care need to be totally aware of what is headed their way.

First, a definition of terms would be in order. "Telehealth" is a broad term that refers to the use of communication and technology to provide health care services – specifically to remote locations. The federal Health Resources and Services Administration (HRSA) defines telehealth as "the use of electronic information and telecommunications technologies to support and promote long-distance clinical health care, patient and professional health-related education, public health, and health administration." "Telemedicine" is actually a subset of telehealth that refers more to the clinical services that are offered through telehealth.

The telehealth/telemedicine concept has actually existed for decades, but now with more mainstream use in the last decade. Why, then, is it suddenly poised to "revolutionize" the delivery of medical care? Let's follow the money.

In response to the Covid-19 pandemic, on March 17, 2020, the CMS announced that the rules would change regarding the use of (and the reimbursement for) telemedicine services. Previous to this date, the guidelines on the use of telemedicine services for patients over age 65 had been more strict. Previously, Medicare's use of telemedicine had been limited to rural patients. Those patients also had to go to designated sites for those visits – hospitals or clinics. Under the new 1135 waiver authority and Coronavirus Preparedness and Response Supplemental Appropriations Act, CMS broadened benefits for the use of telemedicine on a "temporary and emergency" basis – offering (now increased) telemedicine service reimbursements at the same rate as those for a face-to-face office visit. The services could also now be offered to patients in their places of residence. Other types of virtual services as outlined by CMS included "virtual check-ins" and "e-visits." Overall, CMS added 85 telehealth services to the list of those that would be covered by Medicare. Those also included reimbursement for initial nursing facility and discharge visits, as well as emergency department visits, among others.

History shows us that, as Medicare and Medicaid reimbursements go, private payers usually quickly follow – especially when Medicare and Medicaid reimbursements drop. This time it was a horse of a different color, even though private payers were chomping at the bit in the starting gate of the race toward the expanded use of telemedicine. Eric Wicklund in an April 1, 2020 article in mHealthIntelligence notes: "Today's announcement from the centers for Medicare and Medicaid services is a strong stand by CMS, as payment parity has long been considered a linchpin to nationwide telehealth adoption. Several states have passed emergency declarations recently that mandate payment parity in Medicaid programs and for private payers, the latter of which have long argued that they should be able to negotiate their own reimbursement rates with providers." What "the latter" are really saying is: "Here is another service we want to mandate you to use to save us even more money, but we still want to reimburse you marginally for it."

So, the CMS changed the rules and reimbursements regarding the use of telemedicine. How did they propose to implement those changes? They didn't. Instead, they created a "toolkit" for states to use to accelerate state use of telehealth in Medicaid and CHIP – covering over 71 million Americans, including 35 million children. From this toolkit: "Although telehealth services have been available in many states for decades, the recent public health emergency (PHE) resulting from Covid-19 has accelerated the interest in service delivery through telehealth. The purpose of this document is to identify for states the policy topics that should be addressed in order to facilitate widespread adoption of telehealth services, especially when they reside outside the immediate authority of a Medicaid or CHIP program."

It goes on: "States have a great deal of flexibility with respect to covering Medicaid and CHIP services provided via telehealth. States have the option to determine whether (or not) to utilize telehealth; what types of services to cover; where in the state it can be utilized; how it is implemented; what types of practitioners or providers may deliver services via telehealth, as long as such practitioners or providers are 'recognized' and qualified according to Medicaid federal and state statute and regulation; and reimbursement rates. States have full discretion to select from a variety of HCPC codes and modifiers in order to identify, track and reimburse for these services." Another layer of bureaucracy – in charge of implementation. As usual, only time will tell how that plays out.

Later on in the toolkit, we are also told that, "At its core, telehealth is a complex mix of four interrelated domains." The domains listed are 1) the service population, 2) the service being delivered, 3) the provider or practitioner delivering the service, and 4) the technology used to deliver the service. Of course, the "domain" that should be the most important one to patients is not outlined. That domain is: the type of conditions that could or should be treated by telehealth – which would therefore also outline the conditions that couldn't or shouldn't be treated by telehealth.

At least someone seems willing to admit that there may be some limitations here. CMS administrator Seema Verma states: "While not all patient interactions can be delivered through telehealth, our clinicians on the front lines need every tool in their arsenal to fight this invisible enemy."

So, what then are the interactions that can't be delivered by telehealth? These are apparently left to your doctor… er… corporation. Also apparently left to them is the "training" that is to be provided, as the CMS toolkit also makes note that, "Telehealth satisfaction and uptake is also influenced by provider factors such as training and technology acceptance."

When Elinor Burkett and I had our previously mentioned discussion regarding the use of telemedicine, she herself had recently experienced a specialty telemedicine consultation. Expressing concerns that we might be "jumping in headlong before defining the limits," and realizing that this modality would require a "new set of training and skills," she essentially trained herself regarding her part of the interaction. She took the time to do her own prep for the visit, including learning how to position her camera, etc., being cognizant of how the telemedicine consultation would be different than a face-to-face one from her regular medical provider.

◆◆◆

Let's stop right here. As the above outlines, the crux of the matter is the use of telemedicine in its "new age" and the very real concern that patients need to be aware of as the use of telemedicine – in this case, clinical video visits – further expands due to reimbursement changes. To start, let's take a quick look at the historically appropriate use of telemedicine.

Telemedicine has long been used appropriately, and it will continue to be used appropriately in a number of circumstances. Obviously, the use of the telephone is a form of telemedicine. Without getting deep into a history lesson, transmissions of video and medical data occurred as early as the late 1950s and early 1960s. Radiologists were really the first specialists to embrace using telemedicine – as teleradiology. With the Internet in the 1990s came a vast expansion of shared information, and a vast improvement in technology, including home devices to measure bodily functions.

The initial use of telehealth/telemedicine was primarily focused on issues related to remote access. Teleradiology and telepathology did, and still do, allow rapid expert consultation on transmitted information;

and that rapid expert consultation can be invaluable to patient care decisions. Hospital-based telemedicine in psychiatric consultations also started in the late 1950s/early 1960s, with ICU consultations and tele-stroke consultations providing more recent examples of hospital-based use of telemedicine as well as the first telerobotic surgery in 2001. Doctor-to-doctor telemedicine consultations, such as those from ER physicians to outside specialists, are also invaluable, especially in chronically underserved areas. While many of today's proponents of telemedicine reasonably raise the issue of its application in chronically underserved areas, their mission goes far beyond that application – to a world where they see very few, if any, limitations to the conditions they feel can be treated through telemedicine.

Regarding physician-patient telemedicine consultations, there are a number of instances where telemedicine can be used very effectively – especially where patient transport or other issues might preclude a face-to-face visit. This is especially true when a physical examination is not a necessary part of that day's consultation, such as a review of the patient's blood sugars by their endocrinologist, or as an adjunct to help manage a chronic condition, or with some follow-up visits. But what about urgent conditions? What about conditions where an exam by a physician is necessary to establish proper diagnosis and treatment?

I'll answer that question with another question: Of course, if some of something is good, more of that something is always better, correct? Especially if it's cheap and convenient – today's apparent pillars of "good" medical care. And so, we've witnessed an expansion of the use of the medical video visit to cover a multitude of urgent conditions that people were used to getting taken care of in a face-to-face office visit with a clinician – the recent big explosion courtesy of CMS.

Much of the initial expansion of telemedicine was from entrepreneur physicians who, either in their own created endeavors (or as employees of others) offered to treat "almost anything," as we previously noted. (We will assume, or at least hope, that at least this group had some training in the use of telemedicine.) Some of that expansion was from large integrated delivery systems. In 2016, Kaiser Permanente, based out of Oakland, California, apparently experienced its first year in which more than 50% of its visits were virtual visits. I am unable to find data that shows what percentage of those virtual visits were for things like blood sugar reviews or adjunct chronic disease management, versus those that were for urgent conditions. In any case, follow the money. When commenting on the percentage of virtual visits done at Kaiser Permanente, its CEO Bernard Tyson noted, "My model is based on a capitation basis, so I get a set amount of money to take care of 11 million people. I get to invest in this type of infrastructure to allow me to have a big return back to my customers because I am a not-for-profit organization."

So, here we are – at a place where the federal government has further sanctioned the expanded use of telemedicine visits by increasing reimbursements for covered services, and by relaxing the rules on its use. As a result, we will look toward a continuing increase in the use of these services – either by patient preference driven by advertising, or by direct pressure from their insurance carrier. A pre-pandemic July, 2019 JD Power study noted that while 9.6% of Americans had used telehealth services, nearly three-fourths (74.3%) said they either didn't have access or were unaware of telehealth options. The study also noted that "nearly half (48.7%) of responders believe the quality of care received in the telehealth session is lower than that of a doctor's office visit." This, I would assume, drives the advertising push toward "get the same great care as with an office visit," even though that "same great care" is highly likely to come from someone you've never met, or with whom you will never establish a relationship.

So, what are the real concerns patients need to be aware of in the new age of telemedicine? They are the concerns that you will not get the same great care as with an office visit. This has happened. They are the concerns that the clinicians newly providing your care through a virtual visit have not been trained in the nuances inherent in telemedicine visits. This has happened. They are the concerns that your health plan is directing you toward a virtual visit for your condition (even when you first physically presented to a clinic) that may not really be appropriate to be dealt with by telemedicine. This has happened. They are the concerns by physicians that you as a patient may refuse an in-person visit as recommended during a telemedicine consult because you had been told that, in doing a virtual visit, you would "get the same great care as with an office visit." This has happened. They are the concerns that some physicians, convinced by their employers of their role as "stewards of the healthcare dollar," will attempt to provide care through telemedicine that isn't appropriate for telemedicine. This has happened. There are concerns that physician employers will inform their physician employees that a certain percentage (30 %) of all of their visits will be done through telemedicine. This has happened.

Wayne Lipton, a managing partner for Concierge Choice Physicians, accurately outlines "The problem with telemedicine" in a July 12, 2018 article noting: "… the problem with telemedicine is actually much bigger and more personal than marketing or money. With almost 15 years working closely with physicians and their patients, we have learned the most important thing when it comes to medicine and healing: trust. Patients want a doctor who knows them and can be counted on. When patients are sick and at their most vulnerable, they want someone who has been there for them and who understands their health history and lifestyle. Would you trust an anonymous doctor who was seeing you and listening to you via a bad Skype connection to determine whether you should seek urgent care right away or if it's just a cold? What is this doctor's level of experience and what are his credentials? Is this doctor even licensed to prescribe medicine in your state, or will you be paying nearly $100 out of pocket to be told to follow up with a physician in person anyway?"

He goes on: "Telemedicine sounds like a dream come true, but its effectiveness is suspect. You may get treated without having to leave your bed, but what kind of care are you getting? Telemedicine in this form is just the further depersonalization of medicine. Besides, healthcare delivered quickly and face-to-face is widely available these days. There are minute clinics staffed with doctors, NPs, and PAs waiting for walk-ins, and now even drugstores offer clinics where you get screened and tested quickly and then can purchase your medications, all in one stop. Who needs an app? Telemedicine can work effectively in a practice where the physician and the patient have a strong and trusting relationship – the physician knows the patient and their health history so well that both physician and patient can be confident of a video-based diagnosis."

"So," you say, "that whole trust thing is great when I can actually see or talk to my own doctor. And, this telemedicine thing is a lot cheaper than going into the office for a visit. What's the problem here?"

In actuality, many times there may not be "a problem here." Things may work out just fine, especially if you have something like an irritated eye which is mattering, but not painful, and which is not affecting your vision. You may get an antibiotic eye drop and it is possible you will do just fine. Or, you think, I have burning when I urinate and it feels just like the bladder infection that I was treated for last year. Shouldn't be any problem to have a virtual visit and just get some antibiotics to take care of this, right? Perhaps – assuming that there isn't another underlying issue that in no way could be detected without a physical exam and/or lab work.

"Well," you say, "XYZ Telemedicine allows me to drop off a urine sample, and that should be enough to verify exactly what's going on with me, correct?" Again – some of the time that may be true. I have also lost count of the number of times that women have presented to me with vague symptoms and without any of the usual symptoms of urinary tract infection – including frequency, urgency, or dysuria. Turns out, through careful physical examination, that we uncover flank pain and a condition called pyelonephritis, which is a kidney infection. Pyelonephritis is much more dangerous than a bladder infection alone, and some women actually have none of the preceding symptoms of the bladder infection that, left untreated, was ultimately responsible for the infection proceeding up into the kidney. Some women also have the usual symptoms of a bladder infection, and don't feel any flank pain themselves, but still have pyelonephritis. A careful history and a good physical exam and lab work are necessary to sort out the situations.

"No biggie," you say, "I'll try telemedicine first, and if I don't get better, then I'll go in for a face-to-face visit." Again, some of the time you may still be okay. Some of the time, depending how quickly you get correctly treated, and what the rest of your underlying health conditions are, you may be leaving yourself open for a condition called sepsis. Sepsis is where an infection from one part of your body – commonly pneumonia or urinary tract infections – gets into your bloodstream. Sepsis, if not treated quickly, can rapidly lead to death.

Remember, the promoters of telemedicine as a modality to treat your urgent medical condition are not going to drill those safety check holes in the ice (previously referred to) for you. They won't even suggest that you drill the holes yourself. If anything, they will give you a glowing report on the wonders of the unfettered use of telemedicine in an attempt to allay any fears you may have about giving it a try for just about any condition. Witness the following report published in "Next Avenue" on April 14, 2020, entitled "If you need to see a doctor, it's time to embrace telemedicine."

Author Maxine Lipner notes the following under the headline "Novices give telemedicine a try": "As someone who is at increased risk for Covid-19, Barton Colin, 69, is one USC patient who has embraced the technology. With several chronic conditions, including chronic obstructive pulmonary disease (COPD) and chronic pain from a spinal issue, Colin was relieved that he could skip the difficult and risky trip to the doctor's office. 'You watch on TV, and there are six different categories (for Covid-19 risk) – five of them have me pinned right on as very vulnerable,' Colin says. So, when his COPD lung condition flared up, and he found himself gasping for breath, he decided to try telemedicine instead of risking an office visit. Making the virtual visit happen was as simple as clicking a link he received in an email from his clinic. Using his smart phone, he was able to see a tiny picture of the doctor on his screen and the practitioner was able to see him as well. It was a different doctor than he usually sees because his usual practitioner was off that day. After looking over Colin's chart, the doctor was up to speed and ready to help, prescribing Colin antibiotics. The medication helped at first, but two weeks later, he needed to reach out once more, and was able to speak with the same doctor, who prescribed some additional medication."

This is wrong on so many levels that I barely know where to start. Any 69-year-old man with COPD and several chronic conditions who is "gasping for breath" should in no way be utilizing a telemedicine platform in an attempt at treatment. He should be making an immediate trip to a high-end urgent care or an emergency room. Any doctor worth his or her salt will tell you that immediately. The treatment for "gasping for breath" is not just a course of antibiotics, even if that symptom is actually brought on by an infection. If Mr. Colin quickly got better in this situation with a course of antibiotics, he likely wasn't really "gasping for air," or he was just damn lucky. The clinical picture as presented here definitely requires a physical examination and measurement of vital signs, and most likely some testing, in order to determine the underlying reason for his symptoms, as well as to prescribe appropriate treatment. The list of possibilities for his symptoms, given his medical history, is a long one, and includes a number of conditions that might require rapid specific treatment to avoid significant deterioration of his condition.

Yes, there may have been some risk involved in a trip to the doctor's office, but there certainly is no mention here of the risk involved with a "diagnosis" in a complex patient made through a smart phone connection. Jim and Bob's Bungee Jumping/Go-Cart Track/Hog Roast establishment is also not likely to spend much, if any, time outlining to you the risks involved in partaking of their services. So why did you drive past the exit where you saw their sign? Did it appear risky because it appeared "cheap"? A better question: Is your insurance company willing to accept a few "mistakes" for the sake of "cheap?"

Roy Benaroch is a pediatrician who is the author of "A Guide to Getting the Best Health Care for Your Child." His post: "Telemedicine: An Idea With Many Potential Pitfalls – It may be cheap for insurers, but possibilities for misdiagnosis are plentiful," appeared on KevinMD.com. Doctor Benaroch points out the advertising that one large insurance company used for its "Teladoc" services. The advertising noted the story of a young child who was running a fever. The child's mother apparently called "Teladoc" and the doctor "prescribed a medication and plenty of fluids."

Doctor Benaroch responds: "What Holly's mom should have done was called her own child's doc. Depending on the kid's age, health history, and symptoms, it would have been appropriate to either stay home and give a fever medicine, then come in for an exam in the next few days if still feeling poorly, or, if there was a chance of a genuinely serious medical issue, get evaluated right away. The child could have had meningitis, pneumonia, a viral infection or one of a thousand other things. But there could have been no way to know a diagnosis over the phone."

He continues: "What was needed was a risk assessment, not a prescription. Holly's story, to a pediatrician, makes no sense. It doesn't represent anything close to good or even reasonable medical care. A high fever means 'call in a prescription'? That is completely and utterly wrong. So why is Aetna pushing Teladoc? It's cheap. Aetna's payout to the telemedicine company is far less than what they'd pay for an urgent care or emergency room visit. Insurance companies aren't eager to spend money for people to see doctors. Cheap is good for insurance companies, but is it good for your children?"

Despite this, Doctor Benaroch does see a reasonable role for telemedicine. "There can be a role for telemedicine. I see it as a useful tool for follow-ups, especially for psychiatric or behavioral care where a detailed physical exam isn't needed. Telemedicine can also be an excellent way for physicians in isolated or rural areas to get help from a specialist for complex cases. And telemedicine technology is already being used successfully to allow expert level interpretation of objective tests, like pediatric EKGs and echocardiograms. But current available technology – like this teletext service – doesn't allow a clinician to really examine a patient, look in their ears or even assess whether their vital signs are normal. They cannot help decide whether a child is genuinely ill or just a little sick – and that is what parents need to know in the middle of the night. Calling in unnecessary antibiotics is cheap and easy. But it's no substitute for genuine medical care."

So, why do so many physicians – the ones who are able – still refuse to be involved in the delivery of telemedicine? A Deloitte 2018 survey of US Health Care Consumers and Physicians may give us some perspective. Physician resistance to "virtual care technologies" came in many forms per the survey, but the top issue – 36% – was concern about medical errors. Should physicians really be that concerned about medical errors?

Let's examine again who really needs to deal with the fallout when a medical error occurs. Yes, your insurance company may need to deal with that pesky little malpractice "cost of doing business" thing. A large medical device manufacturing firm or large pharmaceutical firm may also need to make a payout from their usually more than sufficient reserves. Who actually suffers? The obvious answer is: patients and their families. Less so, but still in the line of fire, are physicians.

Physicians – good physicians – take an oath of loyalty to their patients first, and stand by that oath. "Do no harm" to them really means "do no harm." And, as I noted in the introduction to this book, truly doing no harm also means "fully attempting to avoid the potential for harm." Physician "resistance" (what corporate types like to further label as "inability to adapt to the times") is often the last defense against the potential for harm. No doubt, it bugs the living hell out of corporations to feel that they can "own" physicians, but not own their licenses.

Corporations have been in the process of trying to "overcome physician resistance" for years, through various forms of "education." Guilty as we docs all seem to feel about making sure the wheels keep turning (see again: "The Business of Health Care Depends on Exploiting Doctors and Nurses"), that "education" has undoubtedly been effective in some quarters. So, the indoctrination attempt continues. A recent "Care Innovations" blog entitled "How to Overcome Physician Resistance to Digital Health" notes: "Citing this 2016 report from the Robert Graham Center for Policies Studies in Family Medicine and Primary Care, the mHealthIntelligence report adds that 'the results fall in line with the plethora of surveys and studies that say healthcare providers would benefit from adopting telehealth – but they're not compelled to use it.'"

Compelled – I love it! Methinks you really do want to own my license, or at least continue to try to coerce me to use it in whatever way benefits you best. Why stop with just plain coercion, however? In an August 2018, article from the Robert J Waters Center for Telehealth, entitled "What's Keeping Physicians From Using Telemedicine?", the authors point to the previously mentioned 2018 Deloitte survey of US Health Care Consumers and Physicians, citing the views of the researchers in regard to the use of virtual visits: "'Our view is that with the changing reimbursement models, growing consumer demand, and advances in digital technologies, virtual care is a must-have for health systems and they will now need to help physicians adopt virtual care capabilities,' they explain. They also called for health systems 'to accelerate the adoption of virtual care, overcoming physicians' reluctance.'"

Apparently we are now way past the point of coercion. Let's just get out the bulldozer. If we just "accelerate the adoption of virtual care," meaning "shove it down their throats," we will surely overcome physicians' resistance, correct?

Humana, an insurance conglomerate that covers over 20 million members in the U.S., apparently has decided to accelerate adoption by making its telemedicine services even more irresistible to its customers. On June 1, 2019, the insurer began offering such a plan, one that would cost employers significantly less than the cost of their traditional plans. Ron Hurtibise, in a July, 1, 2019 article in the Sun Sentinel entitled, "Forced Telemedicine Could Shake Up Doctor-Patient Dynamics" provides the backdrop: "Would you take unlimited 24/7 access to primary doctors via smart phone, tablet, or computer, with zero out-of-pocket co-pays, if it meant you'd have to pay a lot more money to see your regular doctor in person? Welcome to the future of telemedicine, also known as telehealth. Insurance giant Humana is betting many will be happy with such a trade. The company has partnered with a telemedicine provider called Doctor on Demand to offer a discount priced teledoc-based insurance plan it calls On Hand. The plan, which costs employers up to 20% less than traditional plans, became available in Florida on June 1."

Why the stepped-up marketing plan? Hurtibise continues: "Humans, it seems, prefer face-to-face visits with their physicians. That's why Humana's new plan raises the ante. By making visits free to the patient and throwing in most common lab work and prescriptions for five dollars, while making in-person doctor visits comparatively pricey for consumers, Humana, and other insurers, is hoping to compel sick people to consult teledocs."

Later on in the article, Hurtibise also makes note that advocates suggest telehealth will improve access to physicians, given a predicted upcoming physician shortfall. The obvious question to me here is: Has anyone bothered to discuss the connection between a "predicted upcoming physician shortfall" and forced methods of "improving access to physicians?" Actually, Hurtibise does, in quoting Thomas Ferrante – a Tampa, Florida-based attorney for a firm specializing in assisting telehealth businesses, who is commenting on the "requirement " to use telemedicine services: "'It's not a question of if, but of when,' he said. Physicians who are reluctant will eventually buy in, he said. 'It will be driven by market demand. Some will do it earlier than others. Some will be really successful and others, not so much. Some will refuse to change and retire or be driven out of business.'"

Great piece of circular logic here: Let's help deal with the physician shortage issue by forcing physicians to do something that will drive more of them out of business. Obviously, the intent is not to try to keep more physicians in business. It is to control what they do for the sake of insurance industry profits. Telemedicine provides an opportunity for what may be one of the last great efficiency frontiers for those profits – which is, one more way to decrease labor costs. Besides other potential looming disasters, however, an unintended consequence here could actually end up being increased costs brought about by an increased use of testing when an exam can't be done during a telemedicine evaluation. But, never fear, corporate bean counters. If that happens, it's plenty easy to tighten the screws on ordering tests when you have control over those who write the orders.

So, what do these larger telemedicine services advertise that they treat? According to Hurtibise's article, "Doctor on Demand lists the following conditions they [don't] treat: Traumatic brain and spinal cord injuries, chest pain, and/or numbness, vomiting, or coughing blood, lacerations, loss of consciousness, broken bones, severe burns or pediatric ear infections." As I read this, that would leave open for "treatment" conditions such as abdominal pain, shortness of breath, headaches, stiff necks, fever, dizziness, confusion…and, I would imagine, anything else.

So, instead of having an established physician (or her nurse line) you can call to get preliminary advice, you pay your $75 to your tele-doc service to treat your abdominal pain through a telemedicine visit. Depending on exactly what your complaint is, what happens? Do you get reassured that you're okay? Are you told to take 2 tablespoons of Maalox to see if you get better? Are you told to go to the emergency room? Are you told that your pain does indeed appear to represent something potentially serious, and therefore testing will be required? If so, are you then told to go to the emergency room for that testing, or are you sent somewhere for a CT scan to rule out appendicitis? If you are sent for that test and the reading comes back as negative for appendicitis, is the visit over, since an exam can't be done?

Doctors are trained to use a carefully taken history and physical exam to then determine what, if any, tests are required. Remember my previously mentioned appendicitis patient with the negative CT scan? His appendicitis was discovered because the severity of his pain on exam was out of proportion to his eventually negative CT scan. Ah, but what the hell – mistakes can happen, right? Besides, you agreed to that disclaimer at the beginning of the visit – the one that said that the "patient understands the limits of a telemedicine visit." Did you really understand the limits of your visit – or did you still trust that someone else was drilling holes to check the depth of the ice you were driving across? Did the disclaimer give you any idea of the actual chances you may have been taking with your health in getting your abdominal pain diagnosed over a smart phone?

Many of us still have choices – at least for the time being. You are now free to choose to have almost any medical condition treated through telemedicine – if the service is available to you. Doctors are also free to choose to work for tele-doc services, or to choose to offer such services in their own independent practices. Some doctors may be very vigilant in limiting what they attempt to offer through such a service, and some may feel that a telemedicine disclaimer puts the patient in charge of understanding, accepting, and living with any limitations created by using such a service.

Other doctors do not have the option of whether they can choose to provide telemedicine services, as the corporations they work for direct them to provide the service – regardless if they have had training to provide the service, and regardless if they are comfortable with the types of patients referred to their telemedicine platforms.

It's beginning to look like patients aren't going to have any choices left.

Don't bet on it.

Chapter Five What's Worse Than No Diagnosis?

As we noted in Chapter One, at its heart, optimum medical care means care where the diagnosis is correct, the treatment is correct, and both are done in a timely manner with the care being accessible and affordable. Treatment and outcome for the patient obviously will suffer – sometimes significantly – if the diagnosis is incorrect.

According to a study by BMJ Quality and Safety, in the United States a misdiagnosis occurs in over 12 million adults seeking care (on an outpatient basis) each year. That roughly translates to about one out of twenty adult patients. Ten to twenty percent of those misdiagnoses were considered to be in patients with serious conditions, with 28% of misdiagnoses being either life-threatening or life-altering. Another study, funded by the Society to Improve Diagnosis in Medicine (noted in "Fierce Healthcare," July, 2019) looked at more than 55,000 malpractice claims. The study showed that over 70% of the misdiagnoses they examined occurred in the outpatient setting – either clinics or the emergency department – and that over 85% of those cases involved clinical judgment failures. The same article referencing these studies notes that "an estimated 40,000 to 80,000 deaths occur each year in U.S. hospitals related to misdiagnoses," and points to a study conducted by Johns Hopkins University School of Medicine, where Johns Hopkins noted its data confirmed that the number one cause of serious medical errors was an inaccurate diagnosis.

Sounds rough – and it is. Misdiagnosis continues to be a problem in medicine. Why? Despite the fact that our current quiver of diagnostic tools far exceeds those available to Hippocrates, one thing remains constant: modern physicians are every bit as human as was Hippocrates. As long as the human factor remains, there will always be misdiagnoses. And, while modern physicians have been given much more to work with, much more is also expected of us. This includes the expectation that physicians will continue to work diligently to reduce as much diagnostic error as possible, and that they will try to avoid actions that might increase error. This includes exercising caution in the adoption of new technologies.

Sometimes actions that might increase the risk of error are under the control of physicians, and sometimes they are not. Sometimes that quiver full of diagnostic tools can turn on the archer. This, from an article in Health IT Outcomes regarding reducing misdiagnosis: "From the doctor's point of view, the recent increase of large quantities of patient data that physicians must sort through has increased the rate of physician burnout – from the many hours of working with electronic health records. According to a Northwestern University study, physicians now spend one-third of their time looking at computer screens when they have electronic health records (EHRs) in their exam room. This is compared to the 9% of time looking at records that physicians using paper charts spent, allowing time to give more accurate diagnoses and treatments. Additionally, an Annals study shared that physicians spend 27% of their total time with patients and 49.2 % of their time on EHR and desk work. It takes a doctor two times as long to see a patient as it did 10 years ago, spending up to 80% of their time inputting and analyzing data."

How does this translate to urgent care telemedicine? Notice again that I reference urgent care telemedicine. As the earlier referenced study noted, over 70% of the misdiagnoses examined occurred in the outpatient setting – either in clinics or in the emergency department. Recall the top issue of physician resistance toward virtual care technologies – the risk for medical errors. Physicians – those actually using the technology and not just salivating about profits – are well aware of the inherent increased risk for medical error when using this technology instead of a face-to-face visit, especially when an urgent medical problem is being evaluated.

THIS IS WHAT DILIGENT PHYSICIANS ARE CONCERNED ABOUT: FIRST, DO NO HARM.

"First do no harm" is a promise within the Hippocratic Oath that is to be used as a guiding principle for physicians in providing care to their patients. The oath itself is one that newly graduated medical students recite at their graduation ceremonies. As president of the University of Minnesota Alumni Society, I was honored to speak at a couple of graduation ceremonies a little over a decade after I completed my medical residency. One of those years, I decided to speak about the Hippocratic Oath – what it meant to me, and what it may mean to newly graduating physicians. I remember that day well. I don't generally get shaken up in a public speaking role, but on that day I remember being a bit on edge, as the speaking schedule gave me a really tough act to follow. A genius of a man, and a brilliant physician – Dr. Ben Carson – preceded my attempt to provide some perspective on the Hippocratic Oath.

Below is the text of that speech I gave that day. I include this piece of history as a bit of insight into how responsible physicians view the world. To put the speech into its proper context, I'll first offer a short explanation of how I happened to arrive at that particular point.

As it happened, on the day of the speech I was scheduled to have an interaction with a large homegrown health care conglomerate. After I found out how they truly operated, in later writings I lovingly suggested replacing their actual three letter moniker with a new one – "GBL." To some, that "GBL" was the "great big leader" in healthcare – locally as well as nationally. To practicing physicians – fighting desperately to get approval for needed care for their patients – that GBL often seemed more like a "giant blood-sucking leach." As it is, UHC's bite is still felt just about everywhere.

In early June, 1998, I was just leaving an almost four-year stint in a corporate family medical practice. Me – in a corporate clinic? Yes, it was true. The private practice I had joined fresh out of medical school had lasted another eight years and then imploded under the pressure of the mid-1990s insurance industry. I had desperately wanted to stay local and to continue to serve my patients, so I grabbed onto what was available – naïve at the time to the workings of corporate medicine. My commitment to standing up for what my patients needed created a split between myself and the corporation that eventually became too wide to cross, so I moved on. Disenchanted with what was happening in medicine, I thought, "Let's see what else is out there," and responded to a United Healthcare employment ad to see what they were doing. I went on the interview and found out what they were doing. My wife came back to pick me up, and recalls me slinging expletives like a sailor as we drove to the University of Minnesota and I delivered the following address to its graduating medical-school class…

◆◆◆

Distinguished faculty, physicians, graduates, friends and families:

Welcome from the Medical Alumni Society. I'm Dr. Wayne Liebhard, society president, and it's a pleasure to be able to speak to you today on behalf of the society. It's even more of a pleasure for me this year than last year. Now, in my life, I've been cursed at, vomited on, and gotten that "look" from my wife, all scary enough – but at 40 years of age, you would think I'd have gotten over the medical student-like fear that my speech coach could go back and lower a grade on a 25-year-old report card. Even after he did it, I was worried, but... whatever.

Today we welcome you in your transition from medical student to physician and from student to alumnus. We share in your pride and in your accomplishments and invite you to the fold of physicians as our colleagues. That, of course for now, means that for the next three to seven years we will continue to treat you like medical students but call you "residents." Seriously, we are all extremely proud of you and wish you all the best in your futures.

Now, I'll spend my allotted five minutes with some thoughts on our graduates' presence here today, not on the behalf of the Alumni Society, but from myself. This year I can personally share your sense of relief in graduation because yesterday was my final day in an almost four-year stint in a corporate medical practice, after eight years in a private family practice. I know you all had a great grasp of your curriculum, or you wouldn't be sitting here today. I, however, couldn't seem to grasp – excuse me, accept – my four-year curriculum.

What does any of this have to do with you or why we're here today? It's about your oath. In a few minutes, you will all recite the Hippocratic Oath – actually, an updated version of the original oath. The words may be somewhat modernized, but the intent remains exactly the same. So, what is its true intent? I'll ask you to ponder that while I ask you to ponder another question. What really possessed you in the last four years to put yourself through the meat grinder called medical school and then be handed a near six-figure debt for all that pleasure? I would expect at least some of us told the truth at those first medical school admissions interviews, but, even if "I like science and I like to work with people" was just a pat answer, I suspect very few of you chose medicine solely for the potential financial reward. Let's face it – you're all intelligent enough to know that you are intelligent enough to make as much or more money, probably with less effort and education, in a number of other career areas. So, what's the answer to what the Hippocratic

Oath is about and why you're sitting here? Simple – one word – respect. The Hippocratic Oath is all about respect for those whom physicians still refer to not as "customers," but as patients. It's also about respect for those who are loyal to the calling of taking care of those patients and the sacrifice entailed therein. Is that societal respect automatic? Maybe it once was, but it isn't anymore. Are physicians at least partly to blame? Certainly. For example, if we demand an eight-to-five, three-day workweek, and a six-figure salary to go with it, can we expect society to respect us for what we do or chastise us for the money we make? Trust me on this one – we may live in a time where some Americans make much less of an issue with the character of their President. However, they still trust in, and rely on, the character of you, their physician. They trust that you alone will control the use of your medical license and use it to advocate for them. They trust that if pressures on medical practice are extreme, that you will go to the extreme for them – that you will speak out when necessary. Better our epitaphs read "they did the right thing," rather than "they did what they were told to do."

Speak out when necessary. I've been there and done that, and my outspoken manner has gotten me called a few things over the years. The ones that I like to remember are "committed," "caring," and "forthright." I remember those on the days when following through on my oath looked like an uphill battle. Nonetheless, I encourage you to do the same. Whispering about the downfall of medicine in the doctors' lounge and speaking up and doing something about it are entirely different, and the only way you'll be able to do the latter is to really remember why you're here and what the Oath really is about.

Undoubtedly along the way, someone who never has – and never will – come in contact with "emesis," and whose salary probably dwarfs yours – that someone will try to remind you that "this is a new order" and that "physicians just don't want to give up control" and that "our first focus should be to satisfy our 'customers.'" I strongly urge you to resist.

Speaking to this, Dr. Robert McAfee, past president of the AMA, has noted that "the only thing that separates medicine from the trade unions is our code of ethics. That code is being challenged on issues such as end-of-life care, the value of life itself, and the focus on a business arrangement at the expense of one's ethical commitment to do what is right for the patient." Dr. Don Stoltz, retiring from family medicine after 35 years, recently put it in more basic terms in his farewell letter to his patients as he noted, "now every body part can be replaced except the brain. And when that can be done, maybe we can begin to solve the malpractice mess, or even fix up a new enigma called managed care, where all medical dilemmas are resolved by laypeople who have never seen the inside of a nose, mouth, or medical school, and who think your anus is a planet."

That being said, I can assure you that I personally am not anti-corporate, anti-management, or against any ethical means by which to deliver high-quality medical care at a reasonable cost. However, I am very much against the ambivalence created

> when "market forces" and their supporters seek to derail physicians from the patient advocacy that has been ingrained in them by their training, demanded of them by society, and required of them by an oath that makes them morally and ethically responsible. Ethics in medicine, as in life, really can be quite straightforward – even simple – if you choose to remain consistent and firm. Taking the risk of sounding like comedian Bob Newhart, the Ethics 101 course I give to my own teenagers has a simple four-word curriculum: "Do the right thing." In medicine, we have a great guide to "doing the right thing." It's called the Hippocratic Oath. Whether you end up as practicing physicians, teachers, researchers, or corporate administrators – you all will have taken an oath regarding patients that demands your advocacy for them.
>
> So – let's all do the right thing. In a few minutes, when we recite this oath together, let's make sure that we go well beyond the pomp and circumstance value for our friends and family and concentrate on its real meaning – then, let's live it. If we do, societal respect and self-respect will never be in question – and the sacrifices we make as physicians will truly benefit society and make most honorable the lives we lead.
>
> Good luck and God speed.

So, how do physicians best strive to "do no harm?" The answer is really quite simple. We remain vigilant regarding advances in diagnoses and treatments, but we don't allow ourselves to get swept up in trends (more in Chapter Six), fads, or technologies that haven't yet been proven to be safe or effective. Not being "swept up" into usage also includes not being "coerced" into usage – again, not always an easy proposition in this age of corporate medicine.

Physicians carry the oath to bear the burden of "do no harm," not corporations, and they must uphold that oath – no matter how much coercion or reassurance is supplied via the corporation they work with. Notice the use of the word "with" instead of the word "for" at the end of the last sentence. Its usage here is quite deliberate. Corporations – despite their sometimes apparent desire – do not own the licenses of physicians in their employ, and physicians should never allow themselves to work "for" corporations. Physicians should always work "for" their patients. Keeping this in mind at all times will help physicians to avoid allowing corporations to define who they are as doctors.

When doctors express concern regarding the risk for medical errors when using telemedicine, what they are primarily talking about is the risk for a misdiagnosis. The less information a doctor has at his or her hands (with telemedicine, not physically being with the patient to do an exam and order tests), the less chance that the diagnosis will be correct. Desperate times may "call for desperate measures," but desperate measures still need to be adequate to meet the situation. Desperate times also do not change the standard of care that physicians ethically are held to in the care of their patients. If a telemedicine platform is not adequate to meet a particular medical need, then it simply is not adequate – with neither hell nor high water nor a pandemic being acceptable excuses for less than adequate care. (Likewise, in the absence of hell, high water, or a pandemic, other life-threatening issues like "patient convenience" also do not rise to the level of being an acceptable excuse in the event that the platform is inadequate for a particular medical need.)

Consider the tragic case of Amber Isaac. (I will only note the details here as they have been reported.) Amber was a 26-year-old Bronx woman who died at Montefiore Medical Center during an emergency C-section in April 2020. Ese Olumhense reports in "The City," on May 6, 2020: "Though she learned she had a low platelet count in February, Isaac was unable to have in-person visits with doctors through March, McIntyre (her partner) said. Coronavirus concerns meant that the soon-to-be mother was only able to meet with her doctors through video calls, he said, despite her repeated requests for in-person appointments.... Use of telehealth visits for prenatal care, like those McIntyre said he and Isaac had with doctors, has soared during the coronavirus pandemic. They allow a doctor and patient to connect remotely, minimizing the risk of exposure to the virus."

Olumhense continues: "But video calls are not a substitute for office visits, doctors who spoke with 'The City' said. 'We don't have protocols in place for telemedicine,' said Dr. Joia Crear-Perry, president of the National Birth Equity Collaborative, which seeks to reduce racial disparities in maternal and infant health. 'We're building it as we are doing it. So, if you normally, when you're pregnant, get a visit every month – now we are saying you don't need to come in,' Crear-Perry added. 'We haven't decided how often you should come in. Do you need to come in sometimes? Do you need to take your blood pressure at home? What about checking on the heartbeat of the baby? All of those things that we'd normally do in person, we haven't figured out a way to do it from home.'"

In an earlier article in "The City," Olumhense had noted: "When healthcare providers began to take steps to mitigate the spread of Covid-19, the American College of Obstetricians and Gynecologists advised doctors to 'be aware of the unintended effect they may have, including limiting access to routine prenatal care.'" Of Ms. Isaac, she continued: "Doctors induced labor on April 20. That day, Isaac learned she had HELLP syndrome, a group of serious symptoms that can complicate a pregnancy, McIntyre said."

HELLP syndrome is a rare but very serious complication of pregnancy that includes hypertension, and is an acronym for hemolysis, elevated liver enzymes, and low platelet count. It can occur shortly after delivery, but usually develops before the 37th week of pregnancy.

Again, I am only outlining the facts here, as they have been reported, without making any judgment as to whether Ms. Isaac's eventual outcome would have changed if she had had face-to-face prenatal care in the last several weeks of her pregnancy. The take-home message here, as I see it, is that a technology was relied on in a "desperate times call for desperate measures" situation when the most prudent use of that technology appeared to not yet have been determined.

The literature is replete with discussion of the risks related to the use of telemedicine platforms. When the trial attorneys and the insurance underwriters get involved in the buzz, you know that risks are being tied to untoward events. Witness this article from Bronx medical malpractice attorney Jonathan C. Reiter, entitled "Does Telemedicine Put Patients at Risk of Medical Mistakes?" The counselor notes, "Telemedicine relies almost entirely on the patient describing their symptoms. This practice has caused some to question whether the technology is safe. One of the main risks of telemedicine is misdiagnosis. The majority of people seeking medical attention from a healthcare professional do not have a medical field background, which means they might not always accurately describe or identify their symptoms."

Reiter then cites an often-quoted study from JAMA Dermatology: "The study, which analyzed 62 doctor and patient interactions across 16 telemedicine platforms, found that doctors sometimes prescribed treatments that went against the standard of care under established medical guidelines. In the same study, researchers also found that doctors missed dermatological conditions and failed to diagnose problems. Relatively little is known about the quality of the services. A recent study assessing DTC [Direct To Consumer] telemedicine consultations for primary care conditions revealed a lack of appropriate diagnostic testing and poor antibiotic stewardship. Reviews of tele-dermatology services showed failures to collect key medical history and raise concerns about the use of international physicians and advertising prominently featuring easily obtained prescriptions."

He goes on to note some further problems identified in the study, including lack of clinician choice, failure to identify clinician credentials, failure to obtain a patient health history, medication mistakes (including the lack of "basic disclosure of adverse effects, risks, or pregnancy warnings"), and accuracy problems regarding the confirmation of basic patient information.

The lead author of the study, Jack Resneck, a dermatologist at the University of California in San Francisco, has noted, "The services failed to ask simple, relevant questions of patients about their symptoms, leading them to repeatedly miss important diagnoses."

Liberty Mutual Insurance, when outlining their concerns regarding telemedicine misdiagnoses, at least has the foresight to stand up for the appropriate role of clinicians. In outlining their best risk management strategy for an organization committed to using telemedicine, they note regarding clinicians: "They'll decide which staff will use telemedicine, and for which types of injuries/illnesses and which types of patients." Their Chief Underwriting Officer, Jeff Duncan, states: "Healthcare can't be treated like any other consumer service; it's much more important than requesting a ride to the airport. Telemedicine can provide convenience and efficiency, but in exchange, patients and providers may sacrifice quality of care."

At this point, there also appears to be no clear-cut standard of care that state legislatures have established. The National Law Review recently published an article entitled "Telemedicine – Are There Increased Risks With Virtual Doctor Visits?" The author, Michael C. Ksiazek, notes, "As telemedicine use increases, there will likely be an increase in related professional liability claims. One legal issue that arises in the context of telemedicine involves the standard of care that applies. The New Jersey statute states that the doctor is held to the same standard of care as it applies to in person settings. If that is not possible, the healthcare provider is required to direct the patient to seek in-person care. However, the standard of care for telemedicine is neither clear nor uniform across the states."

He goes on, "Miscommunication between a healthcare provider and the patient is often an underlying cause of medical malpractice allegations in terms of whether informed consent was obtained. In addition, equipment deficiencies or malfunctions can mask symptoms that would be evident during an in-person examination or result in the failure to transmit data accurately or timely, affecting the diagnosis or treatment of the patient. Some of these issues will likely ultimately be addressed by legislative or regulatory bodies, but others may end up in the courts. According to one medical malpractice insurer, claims relating to telemedicine have resulted from situations involving the remote reading of x-rays and fetal monitor strip by physicians, attempts to diagnose a patient via telemedicine, delays in treatment, and failure to order medication."

Dr. Dhruv Khullar (previously cited WAPO article) perhaps summed up the present state of telemedicine best when he stated: "Providing medical care virtually is fundamentally different from providing it in person – in ways we haven't examined carefully or sought to address."

So, the practice of medicine ends up at another crossroads when it comes to how we will fundamentally provide care. There are those who will have you believe that the way the steering wheel turns is totally out of your hands.

Don't bet on it.

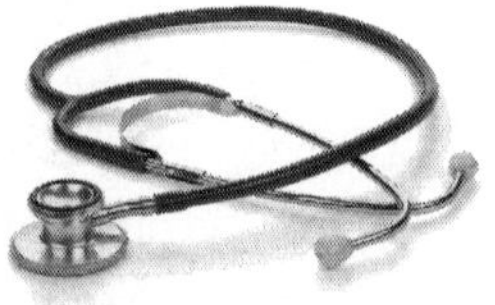

CHAPTER SIX

WHO NEEDS TO SOUND THE ALARM?

Going back to the introduction to this book, recall the statements: "Is telemedicine the next 'fix' in line, or the next debacle? While medical ethicists need to continue to examine the big picture, 'trench dwellers' such as myself need to sound the early alarms. Without these alarms, we remain subject to the risk that experimental trends can lead to entrenched unintended consequence realities."

Is telemedicine really a better way to practice acute care medicine – a way where your dizziness or shortness of breath or abdominal pain gets "evaluated" without an exam and sometimes without appropriate testing? Of course it isn't better – and it carries the risk of potentially being straight up dangerous.

The Covid-19 pandemic, coupled with the subsequent CMS' decision to remunerate tele-visits at the same rate as face-to-face visits, opened a huge door for the insurance industry and its conglomerates. That door, opening into a vast telemedicine suite, was one that the industry had wanted to push wide open for well over a decade – long before the "desperate times call for desperate measures" argument became useful to them. Why the big push? Dare I say "follow the money" yet again? Before the pandemic, the telemedicine concept had already been planted as an incredible cost saving (read: profit increasing) opportunity. It needed to be watered and fertilized in order to grow. Covid-19 did just that.

Then what of telemedicine's future? If the ramping up and rapid increase in the adoption of telemedicine was meant only as a means of providing "safer" care during the pandemic, then – knowing that telemedicine is inferior to face-to face care – we should be pushing for its reversion back to its previous levels of usage, correct? Right…..if the primary intent of government and private payors is to promote the highest quality in medical care. Trust me, I'm not suggesting that either one of these groups is in the business of promoting inferior medical care. And, cost control in medicine is not a bad thing – quite the contrary – as long as the provision of quality medical care does not suffer purely on the basis of increased profits or decreased costs.

It actually appears that both of these groups aren't avoiding the issue of quality with the use of telemedicine. They are instead dumping it into the hands of many they have already tied from being able to do much about it – those of physician employees. As Dr Khullar was noted previously to have stated: "With telemedicine, we've done what we usually do: Introduce a new treatment, technology or care model, and assume doctors will figure out how to use it." Or, in this case, be stuck with it.

The history of the attempts to control costs in medicine follows a long and convoluted path, and knowing that history provides great perspective in understanding just who it is that currently calls the shots. Before a brief history of those attempts, a quick summary of U.S. Health Care expenditures will put them into better perspective. [Chapter trigger alert warning here: A plethora of (very useful) historical information is about to come your way. If you are up to the task, read on. If you prefer to move on to how to minimize the fallout related to telemedicine, you may skip to Chapter Seven.]

Aaron C. Catlin and Kathy A. Cowen give a nice summary of medical expenditures since 1960 in the conclusion of their article entitled, "History Of Health Spending in the United States 1960 – 2013:" "The health sector changed dramatically over the last half century, increasing from 5.0 percent of GDP in 1960 to 17.4 percent in 2013. Over time, the responsibility of paying for health care goods and services shifted significantly, as the household share of spending fell from 56 percent in 1960 to 28 percent in 2013, the government's share increased from 23 percent to 43 percent, and the share paid for by private business increased from 14 percent to 21 percent.

"Major factors such as price and utilization, overall economic cycles, and legislative changes—the most notable of which was the creation of Medicare and Medicaid—have significantly affected health expenditure trends since 1960. Over the next decade, health expenditures are projected to increase at an average annual rate of 5.8 percent between 2014 and 2024 and to account for approximately one-fifth of the U.S. economy by 2024, largely shaped by an improving economy, the implementation of the Affordable Care Act's major coverage expansion, and an aging population."

The history of modern-day cost control in medicine is believed by most to have begun during World War II. The federal Stabilization Act of 1942 had allowed companies dealing with a scarce labor pool to offer health insurance benefits that they could exempt from payroll taxes. During the war, price and wage controls had been placed on American employers, and now, to compete for workers, health benefits could be offered by companies. The beginnings of group prepaid healthcare had already emerged, and by 1950, the number of Americans who carried health insurance had skyrocketed. Penicillin had hit the scene in the early 1940s, and by the 1950s, a number of new medications hit the scene that became available to treat a wide range of diseases. New vaccines were also developed to prevent childhood diseases. Of course, with insurance coverage available, and with new and improved services available, the use of those services increased significantly. This increase in use was followed by increases in premiums, which quickly exceeded the general level of inflation.

The U.S. government entered the insurance business in 1965 with the enactment of Medicare and Medicaid. The 1960s also saw a boom in specialization amongst physicians. By the 1970s, healthcare costs had risen rapidly with Medicare expenditures having quadrupled – along with further advancements in medicine through the increased use of technology and improved medications. By this time demand was so great that there was a shortage of doctors. The federal Health Maintenance Organization Act of 1973 was an attempt to bring some control to American medicine, which was now being viewed to be in "crisis." This was followed by the increased corporatization of medicine in the 1980s, and the continued expansion of managed care in the 1990s as a response to continued increases in costs. So, what were the responses to increasing costs?

Doctor Michael Accad, a cardiologist and internist who offers individualized care in a free market setting, has written a very informative piece entitled, "Why Health Care Costs Exploded After World War Two." In it, he expands on a number of the above issues, and notes: "Beginning in the 1970s, the concept of managed care was introduced in academic circles to provide the government and the insurance industry some models with which they might begin to get things under control. From then on, and to this day, the screws have been increasingly tightened on the healthcare community: price controls, bureaucratic demands, technological impositions, and pay-for-performance schemes."

One of those screws – that definitely bears a little examination – showed up in the early 1990s. EBM, or "evidence-based medicine" arrived on the scene as – ostensibly – another method of improving healthcare. The original definition of evidence-based medicine, or EBM (from Sackett, Rosenberg, Gray, Haynes, and Richardson) is: "Evidence-based medicine practices (EBM) was originally defined as the conscientious, explicit, and judicious use of current best evidence in making decisions about the care of individual patients. The practice of evidence-based medicine means integrating individual clinical expertise with the best available external clinical evidence from systemic research."

Of course, any idea to "revolutionize" medicine – even if seemingly being adopted for the pure purpose of benefiting patient care – must be laid out in such a way that its underlying utilization somehow also benefits cost control, and in actuality, is usually about cost control. The now often-lauded "Triple Aim" in healthcare, as defined in 2007 by the Institute for Healthcare Improvement, promotes: 1) Improving the patient care experience (quality), 2) Improving population health, and (of course), 3) Reducing per capita healthcare costs – all at the same time.

In their manuscript, "How to Practice Evidence Based Medicine," the authors discuss the history of EBM, and its application up to the year 2010, noting: "EBM is often a key component of pay-for-performance programs that reward physicians for meeting predetermined outcomes or performance measures. There is no universal set of performance measures shared by all payers. However, one of the best-known pay-for-performance programs is the Centers for Medicaid and Medicare Services (CMS) Physician Quality Reporting Initiative (PQRI)." (Not surprisingly, what started out as a "pay for reporting" system quickly morphed into a penalty program before it – as PQRS – was officially integrated into yet another amorphous acronym, the QPP – Quality Payment Program – in 2017.)

"Pay-for-performance?" Otherwise known as P4P (no, it's not a Prince song title), pay-for-performance is part of the methodology that payors use to attempt to move healthcare to "value-based" payment. It still uses the fee-for-service system, but ties reimbursement to best practices, metrics, and patient satisfaction. Sounds great on the surface, right? Another great slogan like "Tastes great, less filling." Who could argue with that? Under the surface, of course, things are different. Large payors use P4P to drive your care as a patient toward their ideas of evidence-based "quality." (And yes, that goes way beyond making sure your surgeon doesn't take out your liver instead of your gallbladder.)

Why point out all of this confusing history? To point out exactly how confusing the efforts to "revolutionize" medicine often end up. Despite all the clinical guidelines that have been created, and all of the push that has been made toward EBM, its adoption into healthcare practices definitely hasn't panned out. Why? Ideas that may sound promising at the outset (can anyone say "acute care telemedicine") often end up getting rushed into before being completely examined – and often later end up getting co-opted and maligned.

Hilda Bastian, in "The Trouble With Evidence-Based Medicine, the 'Brand'" (Medpage Today, July, 2015) notes: "Another underlying issue is typical of many social movements – and proponents of most things in medicine, come to that. And that's the self-fulfilling prophecy that comes of believing in the inherent value of something so strongly, that you are not vigilantly assessing its unintended adverse effects. That's something I've long criticized about EBM."

Susanna Every-Palmer and Jeremy Howick give a nice explanation of what has happened to evidence-based medicine in their article in the Journal of Evaluation and Clinical Practice, May, 12, 2014, entitled, "How evidence-based medicine is failing due to biased trails and selective publication."

They state: "Evidenced-based medicine (EBM) was announced in the early 1990s as a 'new paradigm' for improving patient care. Yet, there is currently little evidence that EBM has achieved its aim. Since its introduction, healthcare costs have increased while there remains a lack of high-quality evidence suggesting

EBM has resulted in substantial population level health gains. In this paper, we suggest that EBM's potential for improving patients' healthcare has been thwarted by bias in the choice of hypotheses tested, manipulation of study design and selective publication. Evidence for these flaws is clearest in industry-funded studies. We argue EBM's indiscriminate acceptance of industry generated evidence is akin to letting politicians count their own votes. Given that most intervention studies are industry funded, this is a serious problem for the overall evidence base. Clinical decisions based on evidence are likely to be misinformed, with patients giving less effective, harmful or more expensive treatments."

In discussing funding for randomized trials, they later note: "Firstly, it has become apparent that most of the medical evidence base has been funded by the industry, although these financial relationships have not been disclosed. Between two-thirds and three-quarters of all randomized trials and major journals have been shown to be industry funded. Secondly, there is strong evidence that industry funded studies produce results that differ from independently funded studies. Compared with independent trials, industry sponsored trials exaggerate treatment effects in favor of the products preferred by their sponsor. Although industry influences have been pervasive across medicine, psychiatry has been at the epicenter of much of the controversy about funding source bias and conflict of interest. Among randomized, double-blind, placebo-controlled studies in psychiatric journals, those that reported conflict of interest were five times more likely to report positive results."

Clinicians, of course, are stuck with what EBM

translates to in the trenches as they are trying to take care of individual patients with individual needs, individual problems, and individual circumstances. Kumanan Wilson provides an illustration in "Evidence-based Medicine. The Good the Bad and the Ugly. A Clinician's Perspective." He notes: "… one of the central problems with EBM is when it is used as a cookbook approach and independent thought is sacrificed in the process. Three examples of this include the inappropriate interpretation of: significance testing, understanding the role of chance, and examining subgroup affects. Perhaps the most scathing criticism of EBM is the susceptibility of clinical research to abuse and fraudulent practices."

It is for the above reasons that I chose, as a physician, to sound the alarm when the state of Minnesota attempted to pass further "best practices" legislation some years back. The narrative of my address to the Minnesota legislature is reprinted below, plus a bit of historical lead-in for context.

It is May 12, 2005, and I'm about to address an audience, including the Minneapolis-St. Paul press, at the State Office Building at the Capitol in Saint Paul, Minnesota. I'm there at the request of a group known as the Citizens' Council on Health Care, headed up by a fiery, outspoken nurse named Twila Brase. We are speaking out against the extension of yet another great Minnesota concept in health care – the "best practices" legislation. Following is the text of my remarks – exactly as delivered:

> My name is Wayne Liebhard. I've spent 20 years as a family practitioner in a private practice (one of only 15% or so left in this state) serving the

Shakopee, Prior Lake, and Savage area until this week. I didn't retire. I am leaving family practice to get a job in urgent care work – something that has caused more personal turmoil than I can begin to explain.

I've spent all those years taking care of people in the area where I grew up, delivering their babies, providing their hospital care, taking care of their acute and chronic medical needs – somewhere around 8,000 patient visits last year – people I grew up with, people that taught me in high school, people I go to church with, people who live in my community.

Why did I leave? I left because under current circumstances I could no longer be true to the oath I took, an oath that not only said that I would first do no harm but also that I use all my talents and everything available to me in the care of my patients.

I take that oath seriously. I was given that oath right over at Northrop Auditorium on the U of M campus as I was graduated, and I've lectured about the same oath to medical students as they have been graduated at that same auditorium. That, of course, is the Hippocratic Oath. If I wasn't here today, speaking out against the extension of best practices legislation, it might as well be the hypocritical oath.

To the State of Minnesota as represented here by its legislators, I say: Don't graduate me from your medical school and ask me to take this oath and devote my life to patient care and then tie the hands you've trained to treat you. Don't extend yet another mandate to a growing list that makes it ethically impossible for me to continue to treat you.

Don't get in bed with the insurance industry and its latest "cost containment" scheme. The spiraling cost of medical care does need to be dealt with – appropriately – not with yet another measure that puts yet another roadblock between doctors and patients and again diverts attention from the real issues.

We need to concentrate on what got us here and why costs have risen, and the answer to that is not to give me a cookbook and ask me to whip up the same soufflé for everyone that walks into my office and simultaneously try to force me to make it taste good using only cheap ingredients. Continuing down this road may save some costs for the insurance industry, but when is the last time your insurance premiums went down? I assure you it's not because I'm getting rich. You might, however, want to ask a local insurance executive to explain how it is he took home $124 million last year. (How much healthcare could that pay for?)

Don't get me wrong – I thoroughly believe that you can point the finger just about everywhere – (self-serving) doctors, (non-compliant, oblivious to cost) patients, and (greedy) insurance executives. This system won't come close to being fixed until patients are forced to come to grips with personal responsibility by being forced to come face to face with the real costs of care – costs that they largely engender with their behavior. Something like eight of the top ten prescribed drugs in the country treat lifestyle-related issues – we need to deal with that, but not by "cook booking" our medical care. The public does need to be concerned here (somewhat because of its own doing) about what is being handed down to them. Doctors and the public together allowed the insurance industry to create an oligopoly that promised first-dollar coverage and yanked personal responsibility out of the hands of the consumer. The insurance industry has created its own monster and is now attempting to kill it by unleashing it on the village of Minnesota – with legislative backup. This is a dangerous, as well as short-sighted, proposition – much akin to bandaging a corpse. It won't force people to be in charge of their own health or to become compliant and puts the insurance industry and the government in charge of your health care – neither of which has a great track record when it comes to controlling costs, but I guess the choice is yours – you can have me in the exam room, or your insurance executive. The farm boy in me sees this as the fox being given legislative permission to guard the henhouse, and some chickens are going to fall through the cracks – except we're not dealing with chickens here, we're dealing with people. Let's be honest here – pigeonholing physicians into following who knows whose idea of "best practices" and "evidence-based medicine" will sacrifice quality of care, and worsen the access problem we already have, not to mention the effect it will have on newly-minted physicians in their training and their ability to use what they've learned to "think on their own."

In closing, I'd like to remind you that at some time we are all patients, and patients still expect their doctors will always do the right thing for them – not for "evidence-based guideline #103," but for them. Stopping the extension of this bill is not going to solve our health care cost issues, but putting our feet down here is going to help stop a juggernaut that continues to move us backward instead of forward.

Thank you for your time.

◆◆◆

For decades, physicians have faced unrelenting government and corporate intrusion into the practice of medicine for the failed purpose of cost control. As we doggedly move down the road of continued experimentation with healthcare in the United States, I would still like to keep a positive attitude. A positive attitude for me entails the need to believe that we eventually will foster the right ideals and attitudes – and then act accordingly. In that vein, I will close this chapter with a quotation from an instructor in medicine at Harvard Medical School, also a pulmonary and critical care Doctor at Cambridge Health Alliance – Dr. Adam Gaffney – speaking about corporate medicine: "But whatever their financial future, the advancing corporatization of American healthcare will fail for a more fundamental reason: cutthroat corporate profiteering and the humane provision of healthcare don't mix. As healthcare reform returns to the national political discussion, we should be talking about cutting corporate America out of the health care system altogether – not welcoming them in."

Do we have some answers on how to deal with the new age of telemedicine?

You can bet on it.

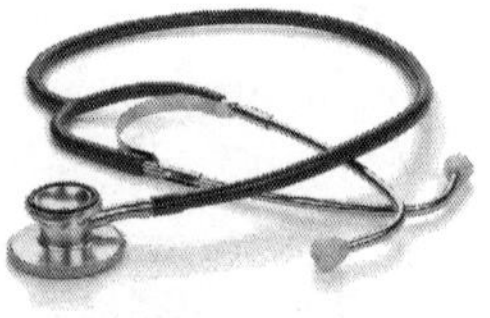

Chapter Seven Minimizing the Fallout

Telemedicine, it appears, has issues – lots of them. So far, I have given you background on what should be considered optimum health care, and who currently is in charge of the delivery of your health care. I've discussed the ever-expanding role of technology in medicine, including the recent boom in the use of telemedicine – its role in cost control, and the risks associated with its use. The risk of misdiagnosis was then further explored while examining the limitations of telemedicine. In the last chapter, we explored various reasons why the increasing corporate control of medicine has impeded your doctor's ability to act solely on your behalf.

So, where do we sit? Where we sit is that – like teenage sex – telemedicine is here to stay. What we're left with is trying to figure out how to minimize the fallout. There are forces beyond our control here – just like hormones – which can drive behaviors that might ultimately result in someone getting hurt. While some parent somewhere might want to install a direct-feed camera in the back seat of their son's 2010 Chevy Malibu with a built-in parent-triggered warning whistle, it's not going to (and obviously shouldn't) happen. While I might want to have a warning whistle go off if one of my patients tries to have his right lower quadrant abdominal pain evaluated by telemedicine, it's also not going to (and obviously shouldn't) happen. We are all free to make our own choices when it comes to medical care, but it is best for all concerned if those choices are well informed ones.

Since we can all choose to make informed choices, we all have a role in the outcomes related to our medical care. Regarding those choices, let's first take a look at the role of physicians in the provision of telemedicine services– followed by the role of patients, and how patients can minimize the potential "fallout" associated with the use of telemedicine. It is important for patients to be aware of the obligations that physicians are held to in general, and here – with telemedicine – to be aware of the obligations that physicians are held to in specific.

For physicians, it is not only best that they completely inform their patients of all pertinent issues regarding their care – it is incumbent upon them to do so. Even though I'm not a fan of all actions set forth by the American Medical Association, the AMA does provide a rather rigorous summary of the principles of medical ethics to which they believe physicians should adhere (and to which you should demand them to adhere).

This includes a section on ethical practice in telemedicine – Opinion 1.2.12 – which notes that "Telehealth and telemedicine span a continuum of technologies that offer new ways to deliver care. Yet, as in any mode of care, patients need to be able to trust that physicians will place patient welfare above other interests, provide competent care, provide the information patients need to make well-considered decisions about care, respect patient privacy and confidentiality, and take steps to ensure continuity of care. Although physicians' fundamental ethical responsibilities do not change, the continuum of possible patient-physician interactions in telehealth/telemedicine give rise to differing levels of accountability for physicians."

They continue: "Physicians who respond to individual health worries or provide personalized health advice electronically through a telehealth service in addition should: (a) Inform users about the limitations of the relationship and services provided."

Informing patients about the limitations of the services provided – for physicians – needs to go far beyond a nursing assessment where a nurse checks the box next to "patient understands the limitations of the visit." Physicians need to take the time in their allotted minutes for the visit to fully explain what might possibly be missed without the ability to do a physical examination and/or run appropriate tests. While it is an important ethical requirement during a face-to-face visit to explain the limitations of examinations and testing (either done or refused) – that requirement is crucial when the option for examination (and sometimes for testing) is not possible.

They go on: "Physicians who provide clinical services through telehealth/telemedicine must uphold the standards of professionalism expected in in-person interactions, follow appropriate ethical guidelines of relevant specialty societies and adhere to applicable law governing the practice of telemedicine. In the context of telehealth/telemedicine they further should: (d) Be proficient in the use of the relevant technologies and comfortable interacting with patients and/or surrogates electronically. (e) Recognize the limitations of the relevant technologies and take appropriate steps to overcome those limitations. Physicians must ensure that they have the information they need to make well-grounded clinical recommendations when they cannot personally conduct a physical examination, such as by having another healthcare professional at the patient's site conduct the exam or obtaining vital information through remote technologies. (f) Be prudent in carrying out a diagnostic evaluation or prescribing medication by: (i) establishing the patient's identity; (ii) confirming that the telehealth/telemedicine services are appropriate for that patient's individual situation and medical needs."

To briefly summarize what we gleaned from the AMA statement: Physicians need to inform telemedicine users about the limitations of the relationship and services provided, uphold the standards expected in in-person interactions, confirm that the telemedicine services are appropriate for that patient's individual situation and medical needs, and be proficient in the use of the relevant medical technologies. The AMA's statement on ethical practice in telemedicine essentially tells us that physicians should use their ethics to guide their actions regarding the use of telemedicine.

How does this apply to patients? You as a patient contemplating doing a telemedicine visit with your doctor may have enough experience with, and trust in, your doctor to freely move forward with the visit. That's great! What if you as a patient don't have that much experience with, and therefore haven't had a chance to develop complete trust in, your doctor. Do you, or should you, assume that your doctor will – per the AMA – use their ethics to guide their actions regarding the use of telemedicine?

I'll try to answer that question with another question: From where do these medical "ethics" arise? There's been an ongoing debate for a number of years on the subject of teaching medical ethics to physicians, with many believing that it is time to prioritize medical ethics education. In agreement is Micah Hester, PhD, Chief of Medical Humanities and Professor of Medical Humanities and Pediatrics at the University of Arkansas for Medical Sciences. In his June 2, 2016 article "What is the Future of Ethics Education in Medical Schools?" he notes: "In 2004, Lisa Lehman and colleagues noted that 'Despite widespread agreement that ethics should be taught in medical schools, there is little formal consensus concerning what, when, and how medical ethic is best taught.' Eleven years later, the Project to Rebalance and Integrate Medical Education (PRIME) group in its Romanell Report (2015) followed like Lehman when saying, 'Despite broad consensus on the importance of teaching medical ethics and professionalism, there is no consensus about the specific goals of medical ethics education for future physicians, the essential knowledge and skills learners should acquire, the best methodologies and processes for instruction, and the optimal strategies for assessment.'"

Lauren Salzburg goes further ("Is the current state of medical ethics education having an impact on medical students?" 2014) when she states: "There currently does not exist a substantial emphasis on the teaching of medical ethics in U.S. medical schools." She further notes: "While ethics education has grown over the last 30 years because of [these] accreditation requirements, there still remain shortcomings in teaching. This is in addition to the number of new technologies or health policy implications that medicine is facing today. Dr. Lawrence Silverberg published an article in the Journal of the American Osteopathic Association that surveyed medical ethics in U.S. medical schools. One of his findings stated that many physicians have found that the traditional approach to learning medical ethics fails to account for important aspects of their moral experience in practice."

Regarding moral experience in practice, she further notes: "It has been reported that up to 25% of patients present some sort of ethical problem or dilemma to physicians. If physicians have no training and ethical analysis of judgment, is it safe to assume they can navigate through it alone?"

So, what ethical training do you as a physician fall back on (to make a decision on appropriateness) when the corporation you work for tells you that "you will be doing a full day of telemedicine" or "30% of all the patients you see will be through telemedicine?" Further, what medical organization is going to back you up if and when you go all Cesar Chavez and decide to stand up for what you think is right for patients? It was the AMA in 2016 that called for the incorporation of telemedicine curricula into medical education, and by 2017, half of all medical schools offered it. Perhaps some of that effort should have been directed toward the gap in med school ethics education – education that could act as a buffer against the corporate "aligning our incentives," "steward of costs," "team player" mentality that may be appropriate in the widget factory, but potentially dangerous when used to guide individual patient treatment decisions over "population-based" ones.

◆◆◆

Let's go back to the AMA statement on ethics in telemedicine, and the part about being proficient in the use of the relevant medical technologies. Amazing how fast someone can become proficient in the use of those technologies. New AMA president Susan R. Bailey, MD, recently stated: "I've heard it said that we've gained 10 years of telehealth experience in 10 weeks as an industry. I think we very much needed a jump-start. We were not doing any telehealth in our practice before the pandemic. And we switched to 100% telehealth in probably less than 10 days."

Ten days! Well, you know, desperate times…

She also said, "The challenge going forward for everybody in medicine is, No. 1, making sure that telehealth services continue to be paid with parity to in-person visits after the national emergency is over. And then, I think, each specialty has to figure out on their own – and each practice figure out on its own – what is the ideal percentage of telehealth to face-to-face visits that's right for my patient population without sacrificing the quality of patient care."

I totally agree with the second half of her statement, and I would fight to make that concept a reality. What I really wish is that the AMA would do the same. It's one thing to put forth a truly decent code of ethics, and it's yet another to truly support physicians – the majority of whom are now captive in corporate medical practices. Given that fact, it is completely tone deaf to suppose that "each practice figure out on its own… the ideal percentage of telehealth face-to-face visits that's right for my patient population…" If the AMA really wanted to support physicians in that goal, it would be spending some of the gobs of money it receives from the federal government (nearly twice as much as from membership dues) to try to do so. You, as a physician with concerns, can apparently remain a cry in the wilderness. (Perhaps it's finally time for physicians to come around to some form of "collective organizing?")

Again, should we be shocked? Of course not, if... you...follow...the...money. The AMA is largely funded by the federal government, which also funds the CDC. Note what is first on the list in what the CDC is telling us about telehealth, as they push for the optimization of its use: "The increasingly widespread implementation of telehealth is due, in large part, to the belief that it will reduce costs and improve access to care..." They are obviously looking for a pretty big score here, further noting the "potential to save billions of dollars in health care expenditures." (A report from McKinsey & Company Health Care Systems & Services has also suggested "that virtual visits could potentially account for $250 billion, or about 20% of what Medicare, Medicaid and commercial insurers spend on outpatient, office and home health.")

Gee, I thought the whole idea behind the push by CMS to further ramp up telemedicine services was to preserve medical care during the pandemic. Silly me... Stockholm syndrome sets in yet again. Kind of like the AMA pushing for telehealth services to "continue to be paid with parity to in-person visits after the national emergency is over." Really? How do we (as the CDC is telling us) reduce costs with telehealth on a long-term basis when CMS is paying "emergency" telehealth visits at the same rate as face-to-face visits? One of two ways, I suppose. First, if costs are expected to go down despite reimbursements staying the same, then it must be assumed that less tests or treatments or medications will be utilized via telehealth. As it goes with the CMS, "less utilized" may end up being a euphemism for "penalized against."

Or second, when the "emergency" is fully over, telehealth reimbursement rates get cranked back down. Josh Archambault notes, in "Telehealth Mandates Hurt Vulnerable Patients And Small Business," that paying in-office rates for telehealth visits (payment parity) is already spiking spending and driving up utilization: "… it makes little sense that policy should mandate the same payment rate, including in many cases, a facility fee, even if the service is delivered from a home office. Payment parity is similar to mandating that consumers at a food truck have to pay sit-down restaurant prices, including a tip and parking. Not only does this hurt the consumer looking to grab lunch, but it can hurt the owners of the food truck, drying up business for their new approach. While not the perfect analogy, innovation with technology changes things significantly and policy should not cement in a one-size-fits-all or the 'old way' of doing business in all circumstances model. One of the driving forces behind the growing popularity of telehealth pre-pandemic was the lower cost to access care. Payment parity undercuts this potential going forward."

So when this all completely shakes out, things may look differently, depending on how telemedicine gets reimbursed long-term. In the meantime, because of everything we have examined, I believe that anyone choosing to utilize a telemedicine service for any reason (sad to say) still needs to maintain a "caveat emptor" approach to its use – unless or until they have an established relationship with a trusted physician. We will explore this aspect more as we now venture into the role of patients as they make informed choices regarding their health care. Despite all of the uncertainties, it is heartening to note that in a 2019 telehealth physician survey done by American Well, 72% of physicians still listed "questions about clinical appropriateness" as one of their barriers to the use of telehealth.

I'll close this part of the discussion with some comments by Judy Hoy, a mental health professional from Plymouth, Minnesota, who submitted an editorial to the July 4, 2020 edition of the Minneapolis Star Tribune entitled, "Online care works, with caveats." She notes: "Although telemedicine has provided critical access to health care during the pandemic, recent studies in neuroscience are providing an abundance of data demonstrating that although online services may work for some, they are far less effective for others. My own practice experience as a mental health professional aligns with the findings from these studies. I worry that the growth in the provision of healthcare services online will continue to expand long after the pandemic is no longer a threat – but for the wrong reasons. Cost-effectiveness ought not trump the delivery of quality, patient-centered care. Let's not treat what science is telling us about the limitations of online care as a trade secret. We need to discuss these limitations with our patients and work toward addressing them as best we can until it becomes safe to engage in-person again."

◆◆◆

Now, let's take a look at the role of patients in making informed choices in healthcare, and how that relates to the use of telemedicine services. I've pointed out that physicians hold an ethical duty to completely inform their patients about the diagnosis and treatment decisions involved in their care, including any limitations that may exist therein. Patients also hold a duty to inform themselves in regard to the choices they make in accessing and utilizing healthcare. The duty of a patient may not be an ethical duty, but, minimally, it is a practical one. Practically speaking, for the sake of you and your family, it wouldn't make sense to go to your car mechanic to get your gallbladder removed – or, conversely, to go to your family doctor to get your radiator replaced.

So, how do you make the choice of who deals with your gallbladder or your radiator? Regarding the radiator, it's fairly simple. First, you go to a car mechanic, not a bike mechanic. Second, unless your car broke down outside of Poughkeepsie (and you, in fact, live in Idaho), you take it to your local mechanic – you know, the guy you trust because you've worked with him before. The guy who is not likely to try to talk you into also replacing your transmission.

Choosing physicians is obviously a bit more complicated. Back in the day, it was said that patients chose their doctors based on the three A's: affability, availability, and affordability. But, as we have already noted, we now have the "convenience" factor to consider.

Stewart Gandolf is the CEO of Healthcare Success, a leading healthcare and digital marketing agency. In "6 of 10 People Choose a Doctor Based on a Convenient Location," he tells us that "Three recent surveys seem to agree; location is a highly significant consideration. What's more, according to Healthgrades data, 'convenient location' is more than twice as important to consumers selecting a physician or hospital than success rates or outcome data. Here are some data points that I recently shared in my marketing talk at the Cleveland Clinic Patient Experience Summit. Many hospital marketers, CEOs and healthcare/patient-experienced pros at the Summit were shocked that people choose hospitals based on location and friendly staff versus quality. Choice of Physician: Consumers who have selected a physician in the past three years are more concerned about convenient location (62%); friendly office staff (56%); than success rates (22%). Choice of Hospital: Consumers who have selected a hospital in the past three years are more likely to choose a hospital based on convenient location (58%); amount of co-pay (45%); than based on outcomes data (30%)."

So, what does this mean, other than the fact that I like to throw around lots of numbers? It means that a significant number of healthcare consumers seem to care a lot more about trust when it comes to a mechanic than they do about trust when it comes to a physician. On the surface, I get that. MarketWatch has already told us that family doctors beat out even Oprah and Tom Hanks when it comes to inherent trust. Inherent trust, however, is significantly different than developed trust. While you might inherently trust family physicians (as a whole) more than you do auto mechanics, you really haven't gained much until you have developed trust with a specific family physician. That specific family physician knows you, and you know her. You continue to see her, because over time she has demonstrated to you that you are more important than the demands of her schedule, or her work-life balance, or any other distraction that could get in the way. She knows you, and she cares about you. You know that if the need arose to do a telemedicine visit, nothing would get in the way of her providing you the absolute best in care – even if it meant sending you somewhere else to do so. She is the one – even if she works for a corporation – that you know will absolutely drill the holes to check the depth of the ice before you drive across it.

Yeah, folks – sorry to say it, but in the end, it really all boils down to you. It's kind of like choosing to stick around during a hurricane instead of evacuating. You do this at your own risk. If you primarily choose to get your medical care based on location, or friendly office staff, you also do that at your own risk. Granted, any physician who removes gallbladders is more likely to do a better job of it than your mechanic, but some surgeons are obviously better than others. The point is – take an active role here. Just because someone offers a telemedicine service for just about any imaginable medical condition doesn't mean that you should use it for just about any imaginable condition. Of course, there are times when circumstances might draw you to the nearest facility – like when the bungee cord breaks at Jim and Bob's. Those times are obviously not the norm. Taking an active role means you actively plan on where to get your care in as many types of circumstances that you are able to envision. An active role does not mean choosing what happens to be the most convenient at the time.

Taking an active role in anything usually also involves making a judgment call of some kind. As my author friend Elinor Burkett accurately points out, a problem we humans have is that we often don't want to make judgment calls, even when they're necessary. Making judgment calls makes people uncomfortable, and honestly some of them, like "how dare you wear white," really aren't necessary. Sometimes, however, judgment calls are completely necessary – like the ones you should make that may decide if you're still breathing tomorrow. When it comes to medical care it is more important than ever to listen closely and ask appropriate questions when they come to mind in order to make sound judgments. If, before your telemedicine visit, you are presented with the opportunity to agree or disagree with the statement – "Patient understands the limitations of a telemedicine visit" – it would be best to disagree. A judgment can't be made until that statement is discussed with the clinician during the particulars of your visit. Get comfortable with disagreement. If you don't, the clinician you are dealing with will make a judgment – that you indeed understand the limitations of your visit – even though you really can't make that judgment yourself until you see how the visit plays out.

So, yes, it boils down to you in the sense that you and you alone are responsible for choosing competent medical care. Before we further discuss patient issues related to the use of telemedicine for acute care, let's briefly look at face-to-face options.

Granted, it is (at the least) frustrating to finally develop a relationship with a primary care physician that you trust – only to find that it seems difficult to impossible at times to get an appointment with that physician – or even one of his or her partners. The primary care access issue is a complicated one, and one that we need to fix. Unfortunately, that will not happen overnight. A large part of the problem rests in the issues that I mentioned in the last chapter – issues that drive individuals out of the practice of primary care, or keep them from going there in the first place. This is why it remains essential to take an active role and have a plan as to where you will attempt to get your acute care in various types of circumstances, as there obviously are various levels of care that best fit various types of medical issues. And in many cases, your primary care physician is now so busy taking care of chronic disease that he either doesn't have the openings in his schedule (or have the interest) for acute care.

The bungee cord breaks after you fall thirty feet directly onto cement, and the end of one of your forearm bones is poking through your skin. You go to the emergency room. You have crushing chest pain or significant shortness of breath – you go to the emergency room. You have signs or symptoms of a stroke, have a seizure, or severe headache/head injury. You guessed it – you go to the emergency room. You have sudden, severe abdominal pain – right, head on in, or call 911 if you aren't extremely close to the ER and have a driver that can get you there before an ambulance would arrive at your location. This applies in any of the above circumstances. The list here is not all-inclusive – there is no such list. Why? Not that long ago (really) your choices for acute care were either your doctor's office (during the day), the ER, or your mother chasing you around with a bottle of mercurochrome antiseptic every time you scraped your knee, fell out of a tree, or were trampled by cattle.

Things have changed. By the 1970s, the usefulness of walk-in clinics was realized, and urgent-care places were born. The earliest ones offered a very limited scope of treatment, similar to what lower-end urgent-cares still do. Around the same time, forward-thinking (?) individuals decided that plain old cars and trucks weren't enough – and we actually became blessed (?) with minivans, SUVs, crossovers, and whatever that thing your sister-in-law drives that looks like a beaten-up tennis shoe. Similarly, forward-thinking (?) medicine types (read: entrepreneurs) decided that plain old urgent-cares weren't enough. They saw the need to stratify (read: diversify). We would have an urgent-care on every corner that didn't already have a Walgreens on it, and every one of them (it seems) would offer a different level of service. And, when we'd filled up every corner without a Walgreens, we'd just put the clinics inside the Walgreens.

There, that ought to do it – no consumer confusion at all. We now run the gamut from kiosks in malls that would offer to do your Pap smear if someone would let them – to high end "urgency rooms," many of which essentially act as small freestanding ERs. What's a consumer to do? A consumer deciding to take an active role does his/her best to find out what level of care is offered by nearby urgent-cares that also accept his/her insurance coverage. It really is okay to simply go to the location you're interested in, and ask. Whoever is in charge of checking patients in can direct you to the right person – on-site or not – who can answer your questions. While I am not a personal fan of drugstore clinics, if you have a mild sore throat or pain on urination, at least you will have a real person evaluate you in those instances. On the other end of the spectrum, urgency rooms and many high-end urgent-cares have CT, MRI, ultrasound, and significant laboratory testing capabilities. Those same ones will also likely give IV fluids, nebulizer treatments, and do more significant laceration and fracture care on-site. They can transfer you to a hospital emergency room if necessary, and also can help provide stabilization before that happens.

If you have a relationship with a medical clinic, or with a health plan, there typically is an after-hours physician or a nurse line taking phone calls for patients with questions. They can also assess the symptoms you present to them and help you make a decision as to the best level of care in your circumstance. Please – and from experience, I cannot emphasize this enough – please listen to their advice when it comes to being told to utilize the emergency room. The urgent-care is not the emergency room – even though, as we have said, several urgent-cares do have higher-end capabilities. If something triggered the person on the after-hours line to tell you to go to an emergency room, it is best to take that advice. It can be quite frustrating for patients (and clinicians) to have to do direct transfers from an urgent care to the emergency room when patients should have gone directly there in the first place. It's not a perfect science, but we should all strive to do our best. This includes those individuals on the "on-call" lines that send patients directly to urgent-cares that they should have sent directly to the emergency room.

What about those of you who choose to use "virtual healthcare" for your acute care needs? Just like face-to-face healthcare, the virtual landscape of direct-to-consumer telemedicine (telemedicine where the patient initiates the care) is stratified. Some examples follow. On the lower end, "Hey Doctor," recently acquired by GoodRx, is an online consultation service providing "low cost treatment over text in minutes" with visit costs as low as $20 and with the promise of providing prescriptions by mail or to your local pharmacy. The list of services and treatments includes birth control for $20, urinary tract infection for $30, erectile dysfunction for $30, acne for $30, cold sore for $30, etc. "DrSays" online clinic offers $35 visits and phone or video visits for common minor illnesses.

"Virtuwell" is advertised as a 24/7 service currently priced at $54 a visit (and even less with insurance), which has you answer questions "from anywhere on any device." Board-certified nurse practitioners form "a diagnosis, treatment plan, and prescription if needed." Virtuwell notes that they treat 60+ conditions, and as is typical of these services, they advertise that their list of services and conditions treated is growing. They also note that their nurse practitioners are in a "profession that offers a distinct, holistic approach that considers the whole person: physical, psychological and spiritual."

I'm certain that this is true about the profession. I'm not exactly certain how all of that happens in an online visit where you answer questions on your device, and then get prescribed an antibiotic. On the walls of the exam rooms of the Minnesota-based healthcare organization that developed Virtuwell are very conspicuous posters with a very conspicuous message. Because of the risk of antibiotic resistance, the posters warn, don't press your doctor at your visit to treat you with antibiotics. Apparently instead, you get out your iPhone, punch in a bunch of symptoms, and then head to the pharmacy for your antibiotic.

"Zipnosis" is also a Minnesota-based company (as I noted in the intro, all the "good" stuff starts here). On their website they describe themselves as a "white-label virtual care platform powering the virtual triage and visits of 51 large health systems across the country." There, a picture of a smiling young lady named Zoey greets you, along with the following message: "Zoey uses her phone for everything. Now she can use it for healthcare, too. Zoey doesn't have time to wait at a clinic. Even a video chat with a doctor is 20 minutes she can't spare. She wants to shares symptoms with the physician quickly so she can get back to her life. She wants a healthcare experience that is simple, seamless, and treats her like a human."

I will presume that, given the chance, Zoey would never use Virtuwell, as Virtuwell notes on their website that their process happens "all in about an hour."

Alright, it probably sounds like I'm getting a bit snarky here, and perhaps I am. Maybe it's because I shook my head a bit too hard in trying to comprehend how the "convenience" battle has now raged into a war over minutes. This is especially obvious when you, as the patient, know what drug you want and need, and just need to convince someone to give it to you. Daniel B. Wolfson notes in the American Board of Internal Medicine newsletter, 7/13/2020: "A rapidly emerging industry has come on the medical care scene – direct-to-consumer medicine via e-commerce. You simply go to an e-commerce platform, describe your symptoms or what you want, and voila! – the prescription arrives at your door, as easy as ordering a book on Amazon. Commonly ordered prescriptions include pills for erectile dysfunction, hair loss and anxiety. You could say direct-to-consumer medicine is like Uber, a disrupter of the normal supply chain that provides better service from the comfort of your computer or handheld device. You trustingly initiate a transaction with a complete stranger and, after verifying the identity of the driver, you feel safe."

Just how safe is that interaction? "Well, it must be safe," you say, "because it is being offered online, and I buy stuff online safely all the time. And I'm young and healthy. And last week I filled up at Jim and Bob's Hog Roast and I feel just fine."

Wolfson goes on: "Can I trust a physician or clinical team I have never met and who will never get to know me and my medical and psychological history? Can I trust that this person is truly qualified – is he or she board certified and up-to-date? I cannot see that certificate or license on the wall. Am I going to be safe – an underpinning of trust? Health conditions that seem simple might be a harbinger of something more serious. If I order a prescription online, who can ask about side effects if they occur? ...Certainly, I would not say that this is a trust builder in healthcare. This approach to care could feed a narrative about finding alternatives to a health system you already mistrust. It could also be part of a wider movement to mistrust expertise, science and facts based on evidence. Today it's erectile dysfunction medication; tomorrow its antidepressants and ADHD medications obtained online..." (Actually, this has already happened.)

That might be all fine and good – and true, Daniel. But, there is money to be made here – and lots of it. The fact that certain medications are prescription in the first place was based on the fact that physician monitoring was necessary for their safe use. No matter – Zoey doesn't have time for any of that stuff – and we shouldn't make her wait, even for minutes. Big Pharma has spent gobs of money on direct-to-consumer drug advertising, and she knows what she wants, and knows what she needs. Therefore, she must have it. She and others don't even need to wade through an online drug menu anymore for their specific medication, as we now have sites such as Keeps for hair loss, Cove for migraines, Nurx for birth control, Hims and Roman for erectile dysfunction, etc., etc.

Medical student Vishtal Khetpal (now a resident

physician) is a freelance writer who weighed in on the issue after finishing a rotation in the primary care office. "Direct-to-consumer medicine is certainly more convenient and discreet than a trip to the doctor's office, where patients commonly endure long waits, only to be rushed through a conversation with a physician who's weighed down by too many obligations. If a doctor's office is like Blockbuster, Hims feels more like Netflix. But I also question whether direct-to-consumer medicine is truly safe for patients. Take erectile dysfunction, or ED. On paper, it seems like a simple diagnosis. In reality, however, it's a textbook example of the complexity of human health. Sometimes ED occurs on its own, with no identifiable cause. But more often than not, is a symptom or precursor of other conditions: anxiety, depression, clogged blood vessels, high blood pressure, diabetes, or hormonal imbalances… The direct-to-consumer companies also present ethical dilemmas. The physicians who work for them may be hamstrung in terms of the scope of the advice they can offer in their ability to follow up with patients to track progress. And they surely must feel some pressure to push their employer's products. The companies essentially operate on islands of care, where doctors can't address secondary issues that surface during a consultation and can't add information to a patient's home medical record."

He further notes that "…the e-commerce model takes the view that physicians are middlemen clinging to an industry ripe for change – much like taxicabs, bookstores, and hotels in the days before Uber, Amazon, and Airbnb." And adds: "In many ways, Hims and other startups are capitalizing on cultural movement. Their products address a genuine frustration with the current state of American healthcare, and they are emblematic of what's likely to be a long-lasting trend toward commodification in medicine." He ends by noting: "I'd like to think there is room for both healthcare models to coexist… But we should push for greater regulation to address potential ethical concerns, draw clear distinctions between health and wellness, and establish guidelines that protect our patients."

Why the long dissertation on this type of direct-to-consumer medicine? This type of direct-to-consumer medicine is still telemedicine but is primarily "asynchronous" (often called an e-visit). In asynchronous visits, information is transferred back and forth between a platform and a patient (not necessarily in real time) where patients log in and provide answers to questions about their condition. Patients can then get a prescription after a clinician or a computer algorithm makes a "diagnosis." These platforms treat primarily lower-acuity conditions, often involving healthier and younger clientele. Despite this distinction, however, Zoey and her friends still remain at risk. And, with the rapid expansion of these and other telemedicine services, we will – with almost complete certainty – begin to see a rise in litigation related to adverse events.

What has mushroomed since the Covid-19 pandemic, and what presents an even greater concern regarding unbridled use for almost any medical condition is "synchronous" telemedicine. Synchronous telemedicine is a "live" visit that uses two-way video, or may use audio only. Its increased use was the primary goal behind the CMS's Medicare and Medicaid policy changes in the spring of 2020 as a response to Covid-19. The CMS's expanded telemedicine access policy for the pandemic again included a number of changes. Some major ones included allowing clinicians to practice across state lines, patients being able to access these services from their homes, phone visits qualifying as telemedicine (with the axing of the need for a pre-existing relationship with a clinician), and the parity in reimbursement changes previously mentioned.

The issues related to the actions taken to expand telehealth in the U.S. are quite complex, and I would refer anyone with further interest to access an excellent article from the May 11, 2020 issue of "Women's Health Policy," entitled, "Opportunities and Barriers for Telemedicine in the U.S. During the Covid-19 Emergency and Beyond." As the article accurately notes: "There are a myriad of telemedicine laws and regulations (that) determine who can deliver which telemedicine services to whom, in what location, in what fashion, and how they will be reimbursed. The federal government regulates reimbursement and coverage of telemedicine for Medicare and self-insured plans, while Medicaid and fully-insured private plans are largely regulated on a state-by-state basis. This complexity in the regulatory framework for telemedicine creates challenges for patients in knowing what services are covered, and for providers in knowing what regulations to abide by."

Wait a minute, you say, the CDC and many hospitals and healthcare centers encouraged me to use telemedicine during the pandemic. Indeed, they did. They advised patients who might have coronavirus-type symptoms to go to a virtual visit as a screening tool before going to the emergency room or their doctor's office for testing. Whatever could be handled by telemedicine during the pandemic was also encouraged, as a way for especially older and more vulnerable individuals to continue to receive care with less risk.

Suddenly, many insurers and health systems decided that they too needed to get in on the action. They started directing previous face-to-face visits toward telemedicine as a further way to control costs. They also provided various financial enticements to their insured members to choose telemedicine visits instead of in-person ones.

◆◆◆

So here we sit – and you need to make choices. You actually have several options when it comes to minimizing the potential fallout related to telemedicine. Before you make any choices, however, you must first be completely honest with yourself. What is it that you really want? Are you primarily interested in cheap and convenient? Are you convinced that you need a particular prescription for something and just want to get it? Do you want reassurance over a virtual platform that your abdominal pain really isn't serious?

You need to be completely honest with yourself, because nearly everything you do in life involves a risk of some sort. You need to be honest with yourself about how much risk you are willing to take in anything you do – and that especially holds true when those risks could lead toward significant unintended consequences. The bungee cord really could break. Those shrimp bought off the back of a rusty pickup truck could land you in the hospital with a bad case of food poisoning. The appendicitis that is actually causing your abdominal pain could be missed without a physical exam and appropriate testing.

So, what are your options?

The first one could be to make the choice to avoid telemedicine completely. How you choose to interact with a healthcare provider is ultimately up to you. If you're being completely honest with yourself, do you want to take the added inherent risks in utilizing telemedicine services for acute care medicine? For you, does the lure of low-cost and convenient override those potential risks?

The next option might involve your utilization of telemedicine services only if provided by and through your own trusted M.D., instead of someone you've never met, and with whom you will likely never interact again. Hopefully you will know best from experience whether your own trusted physician puts your needs ahead of all others (including those of a corporation) when it comes to providing your healthcare. Options you might want to consider if you do not currently have a relationship with a primary physician are concierge medicine, or direct primary care. Both models can provide direct access to independent physicians through the payment of a membership fee. We'll explore the direct primary care concept in more detail later in this chapter.

If it is not your own M.D. providing the care, you do have the right to insist that a physician is the one providing your care, if that makes you more comfortable. In some synchronous platforms, and even more likely in asynchronous platforms, you may not be afforded that choice.

As previously discussed, you can also disagree with the statement that you understand the limitations of the telemedicine visit, and that you (presuming that you are being allowed to move forward from there) will discuss those limitations with the clinician at your visit. Again, if you agree with that statement ahead of the visit, you are telling the clinician upfront that you understand that there are limitations to the upcoming visit vis-à-vis what might be expected in a face-to-face visit. In actuality, it is extremely difficult for a patient to know what those limitations might be without discussing them first with the clinician during the visit – as the nature of the complaint and its possible standard workup (testing and exam) will determine those very limitations when the visit is conducted through telemedicine.

So, what questions should you ask the clinician? Since the telemedicine visit should be held to the same standard of care as a face-to-face visit, I would suggest asking the following: "What would you do if this were a face-to-face visit? What would you do as an exam? What tests would you order?" If you ask these questions (and I think you should), don't be surprised if the clinician – especially in the instance of something more than a simple complaint – bounces you up to the next level of care. Again, I would ask your questions anyway. She may suspect that you are looking for something more, or that your questions suggest you might be holding her to a higher standard of care than she feels she may be able provide in that visit. That's a good thing, as a telemedicine visit should never be viewed by either party as a "way to get by."

You could also ask this reasonable question: "Are you trained in providing telemedicine visits?" To have an optimum experience, the clinician conducting your visit should be trained in providing the visit. When your visit is complete, it also is reasonable to ask: "What could an exam or further tests, tell us – i.e., what else could this be?" If the clinician does bounce you up to a higher level of care, do not resist the recommendation. Do not argue with them that you were told that you would get "The same great care as with an office visit."

Another option is that you could consider accessing telemedicine only for the things for which it was best intended. Things like: diabetic consults, follow-up visits for non-acute care problems, mental health therapy sessions, etc. You will also have less risk in telemedicine use with other medical problems of lower acuity, but again, risk is still there, and the amount you choose to take remains in your hands. Of that, in an AAP (Pediatrics) News article from May 21, 2020, Doctor Richard L. Oken notes: "Physicians have some discretion in determining which patients and conditions to manage remotely. Most televisits in primary care settings are for low-acuity conditions with established patients. Some low-acuity visits may need more than telehealth. For example, most sore throats and adolescents may be viral, but strep pharyngitis or infectious mononucleosis might require laboratory referrals for testing and appropriate follow-up."

As a further bit of advice to physicians, he continues: "If you encounter a high-acuity condition via telehealth and do not refer the patient for an office visit or to the emergency department (ED), you will incur potential liability risk if an adverse event occurs. However, that liability doesn't differ from what you would face if you failed to make a necessary referral following a face-to-face visit or telephone call."

Lastly, if it looks from the beginning that the visit is not going to go well because of poor camera positioning or poor lighting, a crackling audio connection, or an obvious slow or clunky Internet connection – stop the visit. Things likely will not go well, and there's no need to add further risk to the visit. Bad tech issues obviously can occur on either side, and it's up to you to optimize things from your end, including practicing your visit ahead of time. You can also stop the visit if you are uncomfortable with being asked to do things such as a self-exam, i.e. pushing on your own lymph nodes, or pushing on your abdomen.

In "Five tips to prepare for your first telemedicine visit," patients are given ideas to keep in mind to help improve the experience of their virtual visit. These include: 1) Don't let technology derail the visit; 2) Plan for your appointment like you would an in-person visit; 3) Set the scene; 4) Take notes; and 5) Give feedback after your visit. These things you can keep in mind as you decide whether or not you will access telemedicine for any of your care.

Regarding patient experiences with telemedicine, Becker's Health IT, July, 2020 survey of patients who had used telemedicine within the past twelve months noted their top eight telemedicine concerns. From top down, the first four were: missing in-person interaction, technical issues, no physical exam, and low quality of care. The last four were: uncomfortable with video, cannot read body language, not enough time spent, and security concerns. Again, these are presented as issues to keep in mind for consumers of health care as we all make our choices in the pursuit of wellness.

The last three pages of suggestions regarding successful navigation of telemedicine visits may very well get you safely through the process. Keep them in mind, write them down – do whatever it is you do to remember them if you choose to utilize telemedicine. If this sounds rather DIY, it is. Some people are fine with "do it yourself," whether it be auto mechanics, home remodeling, or navigating healthcare. Others would rather find a mechanic, a carpenter, or in the case of medical care – a reliable physician – to trust to get the job done right. As we noted in the introduction to this book, the landscape of medicine continues to change – with some areas of medical care becoming a bit of a minefield – requiring pertinent background information for safe navigation. We've pointed out the risks associated with that navigation.

As a consumer of medical care, you can again choose to DIY that navigation, or find someone reliable to do it for you. In the not so distant past, it wasn't all that difficult to find that reliable someone. Your family doctor or other primary care provider (internist or pediatrician) was the person you could trust. In the not so distant past, they were likely to be members of private (not corporately owned) clinics where their loyalty was single (to you) – and not dual (to you and their large corporate employer).

Fast forward to the present. As we noted in the intro, as of 2018, less than one third of medical practices in the United States remained private. So, in the present, it's not all that easy to go out and find a primary care physician that is still in private practice – especially in a state like Minnesota, where the numbers are worse than the national average.

Before we go any further, it is important – and fair – to note that there are many primary care doctors who work in large medical corporations who are continuously as solid and as ethical as the day is long. They are also typically under a lot of pressure from their corporate employers, as we have already pointed out. So, as a consumer of medical care, is there an alternative to corporate-run medical care?

The answer is yes. Despite their dwindling numbers (as we have pointed out), traditionally run independent medical clinics do still exist, but are becoming increasingly harder to access. Another option, as mentioned earlier, is known as direct primary care – an independent option which can also have financial advantages for patients. Who better to explain the concept of direct primary care (DPC) than one of its practitioners?

With this in mind, I consulted Dr. Don Gehrig, an internal medicine physician who has been in practice in the Twin Cities for 41 years, and who eight years ago decided to go the route of direct primary care. I posed a number of questions to him about the nature of direct primary care as well as the advantages of this model for patients in today's medical environment, and I very much appreciated Dr. Gerhig's straightforward answers to my questions. There is no room anymore in the discussion of today's provision of healthcare for anything other than brutal, straightforward honesty – and Dr. Gehrig held nothing back in his opinions regarding today's healthcare environment.

As an answer to my first question regarding the advantages of DPC for the patient in today's medical environment, Dr. Gehrig noted: "The main advantage for patients in finding and choosing a DPC doctor is that they indeed have a personal physician, not just a provider. Someone who works for them personally, directly – i.e., a true professional relationship – a rarity in medicine this whole century." He went on: "Primary care doctors in managed-care organizations do not work for patients – they work for their employer. Essentially, they work for RVUs [relative value units] which is how they're paid. There are mere 'providers,' making and manufacturing billable RVUs for their multibillion-dollar non-physician employers, while avoiding penalty or clawbacks for that employer – and did I mention patient or physician in that essential descriptive?"

My next question involved the workings of DPC, including payments. Dr. Gehrig noted: "In my DPC, the predominant payment style I use is FFS (fee for service). I bill so many dollars per 10 minute intervals, like lawyers or accountants. Each lab drawn has a price based on my costs and small markup for the real extra time of drawing, handling, lab service contracting, interpreting and delivering back to the patient that additional result. Some of my patients with more complexity have preferred a package for the whole year, having needs for more frequent visits or testing, such as warfarin or diabetic patients. That price usually gives them a 10 to 20% discount for the year. I also have a one lump sum for the year for my few LTC (long-term care) patients, which has always generated lots of nursing home visits and tons of weekly phone calls, faxes and orders to sign. My one fee for the year [for them] covers my fees, office calls, physicals, pre-ops, phone calls-texts-emails-prior authorizations, refills and labs done through my business' tax ID #. It does not cover outside imaging, outside consultations, procedures or hospitalizations. Basically all of my patients get 'concierge' like access to me as a solo doctor with a tiny bureaucratic framework supporting me (the art of small, as I call it)."

I moved on to ask about the types of problems that a DPC physician might address through telemedicine. Dr. Gehrig's response: "I've had no reason whatsoever to do the laborious HIPAA proof highly bureaucratized and televised 'telehealth visit.' I use the T E L E P H O N E [emphasis is his] – it's been around for over 100 years, and still works fine. Then I document the call in my chart – every time. Have for 41 years. The 'telehealth visit' craze has become necessary for these 'too big' clinics which have huge viral infested waiting rooms most of the year, but can still generate revenue so their 'too big' clinics don't just up and die. Then, somehow call that 'care' is quite a stretch. AND, it is still only operating under EUA reimbursement executive orders from President Trump, during this pandemic crisis."

I then posed the question: "What do patients like most about DPC?" Dr. Gehrig: "Patients like the access and also no billing BS. In my 41 years of patient care, they didn't like third-party billing crap anymore than we do or did! They have a reliable respondent, clinical touchstone – a personal physician! There's that phrase again." He also noted: "My long-term ethic has been that the only ethical 'single payer' should be our next patient, otherwise who does one truly work for?"

One of my final questions was about the types of control that corporations have over physicians. Regarding his own experience, Dr. Gehrig commented: "I said no 8 years ago. But I am probably the last IM (internal medicine physician) here to do this. Our time is past. We were the sick patient doctor of the late 1950s to the early 2000's era of medicine. We were trained in the art and practice of taking care of the dying heart patient, in and out of the hospital the last 10 years or so, after your first MI (heart attack) was defended, not ever interrupted. And that fortunately isn't happening, as it once was so – which is a good thing! We've sort of been relegated to the Maytag repair man status. We're evolving into a very impersonal and distant sort of system of delivery, and in some ways, our great endothelial stabilizers (heart medications) have afforded this great transformation, so long as you can get access to them, somehow."

He also noted: "Divided loyalties between coding, billing and maximizing RVUs, and those true needs of the next patient cannot be done without sacrificing one's sworn patient allegiances, in my opinion. In my near 50 year experience spanning many big government intrusions, my simpler direct pay patients have given me my professionalism back – patients get it very quickly."

◆◆◆

Again, I appreciate the fact that Dr. Gehrig was very straightforward with his opinions, and with his answers to my questions. As he accurately points out, the traditional practice of internal medicine is fading, but it does actually appear now that more and more physicians are choosing the DPC route – so that bodes well for the future availability of independent clinicians.

The fact is – no matter how you ultimately choose to access your care, the degree of trust between you and your clinician is the most important factor in the success of your relationship. It is essential that you are comfortable with your clinician's style of practice and with his or her commitment to your well-being. Developing this level of trust can also further assure you that factors outside of the doctor-patient relationship will not be allowed to have an adverse effect on your care.

There is no doubt that the landscape of healthcare is changing rapidly, and will continue to do so. Greek philosopher Heraclitus eloquently addressed the concept of change when he quipped, "change is the only constant in life." As consumers of health care, we need to remain ready to deal with constant changes. Our assignment is to keep a close watch on the highway ahead of us – to know what's coming our way in order to appropriately react, and to avoid getting run over.

Godspeed to us all!

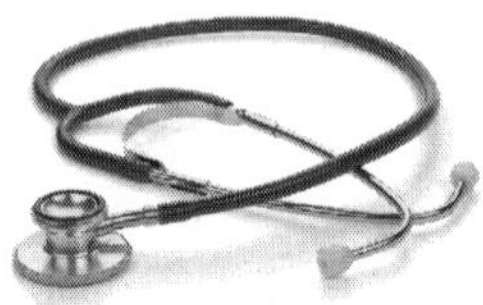

Appendix Further Exploration: Health Care Costs

Since I started medical school in the fall of 1979, it seems that the medical profession has been constantly peppered with the "cost of medical care" issue. Cost had been debated as an issue much earlier, but the 1970s saw significant policy changes in an attempt to control costs. Of course, the cost issue is intimately tied to the subject of telemedicine, as we have pointed out throughout this book. I also rigorously tackled the issue of cost throughout "Elephants in The Exam Room – The Big Picture Solution Today's Health Care 'Crisis,'" which I wrote in 2009. At the end of this section are some cost statistics from the beginning of that book. I've included them here because the sad fact is that while the cost numbers have changed – upwards – nothing else really has. More up-to-date stats have also been added next to the old ones for comparison. The frustration continues as the corporate control of medicine increases while reform of the true drivers of healthcare costs never seems to materialize.

Somehow the powers that be are still convinced that allowing further corporate control of medicine (now add telemedicine) will translate into cost savings

– savings that will be passed on to the consumer. You'd think they would've learned by now. That last sentence is, of course, the fallacy in this kind of thinking. That fallacy is the presumption that someone is actually being duped here, versus today's reality of a much more complicit approach to policy. The shell game continues, and doctors continue to be blamed for high costs because they don't provide "quality" care. This is despite having to deal with the large segment of our population that is obese and/or noncompliant with treatment recommendations (non-compliance estimates run at around 50%). This group often develops the chronic diseases that account for 75% of our total health care costs. Despite the obvious, medical "outcomes" somehow get directly correlated with "quality" of care, and the cycle continues.

While pundits rave about the ability of other countries to contain healthcare costs, they also seemingly overlook the 5% of our population that consumes half of our health care dollars. In many of those countries, that "5% of the population" would not receive the kind of care – and therefore generate the kind of costs – that they do here. It remains much easier to blame "poor quality" care for our cost issues, rather than looking at reality – including the massive amount of money we spend on "health maintenance" for lifestyle-related conditions, instead of just plain "health care."

See the next pages for cost statistics (and their updates) from "Elephants in the Exam Room."

Why does health care cost so much?

Facts:

• 2007 health care spending was $2.2 trillion which equaled 6.2% of our GDP. (2018: 3.6 trillion/17.7% GDP)

• 30% of our health care dollars are being spent on about 1% of our population. (2016: 22% of our health care dollars.) [On the other side of the coin: 50% of the population currently accounts for only 3% of healthcare spending.]

• 50% of all health expenditures are spent on the 10 most expensive medical conditions, and 5% of patients account for nearly half of all health care expenditures in a given year, as noted in "In Brief," in the July 11, 2005 edition of American Medical Association News. (2016: 5% of population still accounted for half of healthcare spending.)

• Eight of the top ten prescribed drugs treat problems tied primarily to lifestyle. (Primarily still true.)

• Roughly two-thirds of American adults are overweight. (About half of these are now considered "obese".)

• It has been estimated that around 40% of the total cost of health care is spent on administration. (2020: 34.2%, but still the highest administrative costs of all advanced countries.)

• Bill McGuire, CEO of United Healthcare, made $124.8 million total compensation in 2004 and sat on $1.6 billion in stock options in 2006. (Great strides here: New CEO David Wichmann took home only $52 million in 2019.)

• General Motors estimates that $1500 of the cost of every vehicle it produces in the U.S.results from the cost of providing health care to its employees. (At GM, annual health care expenditures rose from $665 million in 2011 to more than $1 billion currently.)

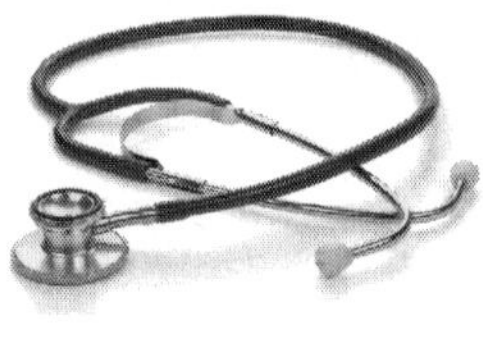

THE "MINNESOTA EXPERIENCE"

(OR—HOW CORPORATE CONTROL OF AMERICAN MEDICINE TOOK ROOT)

The AMA released a study as far back as 2006 noting that health-plan market domination of medical care in the U.S. was, by then, virtually complete. In the May 8, 2006 issue of American Medical News, Bob Cook, in fact, wrote an article entitled, "AMA study: Health plan market domination virtually complete." He noted: that "…in just about every metropolitan area, one or two firms controlled at least half of the HMO/PPO market." What did that mean? It meant that by then, just a few health plans overwhelmingly dominated the market in almost every area of the country. Why? As Cook reported, in the twelve previous years, there had been more than 400 health-plan mergers. Mega-health plans have long touted that mergers reduce overall costs, and that this somehow translates into lower premiums to consumers. Apparently, that magical thinking somehow also kept the Justice Department off their backs, which seems to have worked, in that conditions apparently were placed on only two of those over 400 mergers. Meanwhile, physicians still aren't allowed to bargain collectively.

So, mega-health gets increasingly mega, but instead of passing the savings on to you, it is handsomely paying its board, who then handsomely rewards its CEO with $1.6 billion in stock options (something that likely wouldn't happen if all of healthcare were regulated profit or not-for-profit).

The insurance industry (auto, home, life, disability, health) never loses money in the aggregate. It doesn't have to. It either raises premiums or changes the conditions in its policies based on the experiences of its coverage groups. Should the insurance industry lose money? No. It's a business that is supposed to insure you against huge losses – losses which you couldn't otherwise pay. As regards health care, should it continue to post record profits while continuing to increase premiums on a yearly basis? Why not? We seem to be unwilling to limit its absolute takeover of the health care industry – we actually foster it. Does the auto insurance industry or the homeowners' insurance industry have this much control over repair shops and building contractors? How did we get here, anyway?

The Minnesota experience is a perfect example of how we got here, and explains what has been coming your way for years, and what else may be on the way. Our answer here for the problems we saw in health care was to put the insurance industry in charge. Minnesota – the birthplace of Paul Bunyan, Charles Lindbergh, and the HMO. To further understand why physicians, and therefore you as the patient, have so much restriction (i.e. so little control) at this point, we'll take a brief recall of history as it applies to the current climate.

Minnesota Physician magazine captured the essence of our march to managed care back in July, 1998 in an article by Gerald F. Moran, F.A.C.M.P.E., and Robert E. Thompson entitled, "How We Got There – A Brief History of Managed Care in the Twin Cities." It opens: "'The Minnesota Experience' is a catchphrase for America's swift march into health maintenance organizations (HMOs). Although they did not anticipate managed care as we know it today, it was big Twin Cities corporations and physician leaders that led the charge. In the early 1970s, hospitals and physicians were denounced as cottage industries, and were said to be too passive about out-of-control costs. But by early 1998, Corporate Report was describing Twin Cities health care as "three health plans dominating to the point of oligopoly."

It goes on: "In 1970, Paul Ellwood, a Minneapolis pediatric rehabilitation specialist and aspiring health policy expert, coined the term 'health maintenance organization.' Ellwood penned an article for Fortune magazine envisioning a marketplace of corporate-style organizations financing and delivering prepaid benefits through a multispecialty staff of employed physicians. President Richard Nixon seized on the concept, proposing to Congress in 1971 a national HMO strategy to convert American doctors into competitors vying for customers on the basis of quality and price. Federal enabling legislation quickly followed and by 1976 the Twin Cities supported 6 HMOs, whose 141,000 members represented almost 6 percent of the metro area population."

And the rest is history.

As my own history goes, if United Healthcare was my personal last chance of owning my own island, then my Paul Ellwood connection was probably the first. It is late June, 1983, and I'm preparing to start my medical internship in St. Paul. Unsure at that time if I really want to commit myself completely to the practice of medicine forever, and full of broader ideas, I interview with Paul Ellwood, who is looking for new staffers. By then, Paul had established a think tank named "Interstudy," located in Excelsior, Minnesota, and I visited him there. Of course, I didn't join on, and went on to the internship, etc., etc. As was the case at United Healthcare, my wife dutifully accompanied me, knowing full well ahead of time what would happen.

One of Paul's staffers, Richard Burke, did go on to be able to afford his own island, and as so often happens, history becomes circular here. In 1973, the Hennepin County Medical Society in the Twin Cities decided to set up its own HMO and named it PHP (Physicians' Health Plan), and contracted Richard Burke to provide the management services. Unfortunately, the plan wasn't run tightly enough, didn't do well financially, and also drew the ire of the Federal Trade Commission.

The PHP board essentially turned the whole operation over to Burke, who used it to create a publicly-traded management company. Burke and others reaped enormous gain from their shares in the management company, which eventually became – sound the trumpets – United Healthcare.

It is really quite interesting for me to think – almost forty years later – about how the world could have changed for me if I would have decided to become one of Paul Ellwood's staffers. This, instead of following through with an internship and Family Practice residency, and now almost forty years of births and deaths and nights and weekends and triumphs and tears and fighting to maintain a constantly threatened profession...which I'm damn glad I did . As I have discovered over the years, nearly every doctor I know understands the frustration of dealing with some corporate types who – even with a gun held to their heads – couldn't muster the guts it takes to attend to a critical patient. That reward alone keeps many of us sane as we continue to work toward some semblance of balance between corporate demand and the doctor-patient relationship.

To every principled doctor who is reading this: Thank you for what you do, what you have done, and what you will do. There is no amount of money, or any 15th floor corner office that will ever come close to equaling the benefit of what you do for those you take care of – or to equaling the guts it took to endure the training of becoming a physician. My eternal admiration to each and every one of you!

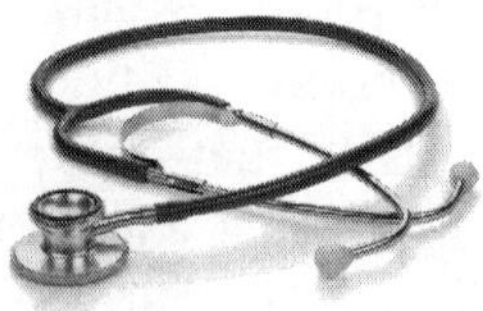

About the Author

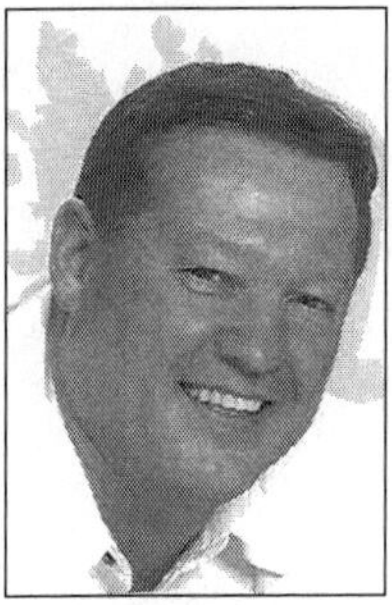

Wayne Liebhard, MD, a Minnesota native and family physician for twenty years, now practices in an emergency medicine clinic. He has won numerous national awards as an author and songwriter, gaining special acclaim for his book *Elephants in the Exam Room—The Big Picture Solution to Today's Health Care "Crisis,"* (2009) and music from the album *Here—In Flyover Country*.

Besides his doctorate from the University of Minnesota and residency at St. John's Hospital (St. Paul), he holds undergraduate degrees in the natural and social sciences from Saint John's University (Minnesota). He has consistently advocated for the sanctity of the doctor-patient relationship, and his articles have appeared in numerous publications ranging from "Minnesota Physician" to "Mustang Monthly."

He lives in Minnesota with his wife, Joy, and his Ford Mustangs. His classic rock band is still cranking out the tunes and releasing new music albums and music videos.